Praise for *Life after Prostate Urological Surgeries: 10 Weeks from Incontinence to Continence—Vanita's Way*

Post-Prostatectomy

I was referred to Vanita by my urologist following prostate surgery. In a matter of a few weeks I regained control of my bladder and left the pads behind. Vanita has a straightforward approach to therapy, founded on experience and common sense. She has a proven track record, and I am grateful for her guidance.
-Richard F., 70 years young

I started seeing Vanita about a week after my surgery. After a couple of weeks of her program I was only using small pads. Within 9 weeks I was not using any pads, Vanita's program helped me get back to a normal life. Thank you, Vanita.
-Ronald G. 52 years old

At the urologist's request, Vanita visited me while I was in hospital after a Radical Prostatectomy. She provided hope, and later in her gentle way, enabled me to regain control of bladder function. Now, over two years since surgery after the cancer returned, requiring Radiation Therapy in the area of the urethra and bladder, Vanita helped me again to successfully attain bladder control.
-Riley L. 70 years old

I am deeply thankful to Vanita for her help in overcoming my discomforts resulting from prostate medical procedures. My wife, Dorothy, sat in and listened to her instruction, especially the nutritional guidance, and also did all of the daily exercises that Vanita had assigned as therapy for me. She, too, has found that Vanita's instruction and the performance of the exercise have greatly relieved her of modest incontinence. I have not had to use a pad since my last visit with Vanita. I am faithful in performing my therapy exercises as Vanita has prescribed. Thank you!
-Jim B.

*I had Robotic Prostatectomy on November 9th 2012. My catheter was removed 4 days later on November 13th. I started my visits to Vanita's rehab on Thursday November 15th. I returned to work on January 3rd dry and using no pads. My rehab took about 6 weeks and was very successful. I still do many of the exercises that I was taught at Vanita's to maintain my level of continence and confidence. I did not always understand why some of the exercises worked, but Vanita would explain the reason and importance of each activity as we moved through the progression from large pads to thin pads to no pads. **This experience has taught me that an expert in a field can help you much more than trying to figure it out on the internet by yourself.** Several patients who had their surgery at the same time as me, struggled because they tried to do it on their own. They were still working on their continence long after I was dry and back to the job. I referred them to Vanita and they improved after just one visit and were able to regain full continence in less than 6 weeks. Vanita helped me get my life back to normal and I thank her for that. She is the #1 expert in the Melbourne area and has now taken on a large number of patients from Orlando and around the state. I have also recommended her to two on my co-workers, and they had similarly successful results.*

-Derik E.

It is with great pleasure to say that with Vanita's help and her therapy, I am myself again. I had given up on life after surgery, but with Vanita's encouragement and the quick results of the therapy I can now live a normal life again. I can highly recommend Vanita to anybody having prostate surgery. Life for me is great again after the therapy and exercises I received at her office.

-Walter E., 74 years old

As a former professional martial arts instructor, I was used to training very hard in all physical activity, the exact opposite of what was needed to successfully deal with the after effects of prostate surgery. Vanita exhibited extreme patience and was very understanding in helping me through this most challenging time. I am eternally grateful to her for her untiring efforts to help me physically, mentally and emotionally deal successfully with my prostate removal surgery.

-Ron K., 72 years old

"Vanita's knowledge, practical expertise, and sunny personality facilitated and expedited my recovery from prostate surgery."
-James W., 73 years old

"I wish to express my thanks for the support you have provided during my recovery from prostatectomy. Your advice and exercises have been most beneficial."
-David O.

"I want to thank you for everything you've done to speed up the healing process after my surgery. Without your guidance, encouragement, and support I never would have accomplished so much in so little time. I'm forever grateful to you for all you have done."
-Jim M.

"Vanita, you never cease to amaze me with your thoughtful generosity. Thank you so much for your kindness and conversations. It is so comforting to know that we are all going through some of the same problems."
-John C.

FEMALES

My experience with Vanita was very positive. She is a loving and caring individual. I am still doing the exercises that she taught me to do and they have helped immensely. I learned from Vanita how important it is to do the exercises correctly. I am doing very well at this time and am thankful that Vanita is there for so many people in our community.
-MJH, 72 years old

I was referred to Vanita due to my severe issues with regard to my pelvic floor. Vanita impressed me with her knowledge of my problem, and after two sessions a week over three weeks I started noticing some relief, and after our five weeks of treatment I was completely back to my normal. Thank you, Vanita; you are an Angel to me!
-Susan D.

I was a little unsure as to what to expect when Vanita was recommended to me by my doctor, but she quickly put me to ease, and I felt right at home during my visits. With the home exercises she gave me, and my weekly visits with in-office treatment, I was able to overcome the issue I was having and I'm now symptom free! Thanks so much Vanita!
-Sue L.

I pride myself on being healthy, active and in control of my life, but episodes of little "accidents" from incontinence eroded that self-image. When I finally went to a urologist to "do something" about my old-lady bladder, he examined me, said the bladder was perfectly healthy and that I should try everything else before resorting to medication. That suited me because another pill in my life was not welcome. However, his referral for therapy seemed like a long shot. After all, I knew the Kegel exercise from childbirth classes 40 years ago and it didn't seem to work. Vanita's cheerful, persistent, and logically explained exercises, both physical and especially mental, made an immediate impact on my control issues. Six weeks later my confidence had returned, along with a degree of control I thought was lost forever. No more embarrassing dashes to the bathroom or soiled underwear, and a new and welcome awareness of my own body. I will always be grateful that Vanita became a part of my life.
-Marilyn F., 72 years old

My urologist referred me to Vanita before resorting to surgery. Vanita's therapy was successful and I am very happy with the results. Vanita is very friendly and the sessions are not stressful. She gives lots of advice and makes you feel confident about your progress. Thank you for your help, Vanita!
-Pat W., 74 years old

I went to Vanita's Rehab for my incontinence. At the time I had a padded bed and wore a diaper. After therapy with Vanita I only had to wear a panty liner. On top of that, Vanita is very sweet.
-Emily E., 90 years old

"Vanita, dear! That's what you have become, a dear friend! The therapy that you and my husband worked together on has proven to be a great success! It's sad to see him "graduate" from your therapy program. We shall miss you and your loving ways! We shall recommend you to all who have this

problem; they too, if they work at it, will have the same success. With love, gratitude, and a big hug..."
-Diane on behalf of Allen B., 89 years old

"Thank you so much for all of your help before we went on our trip. I'm doing very well and following your instructions. It is wonderful living with my family, and your help made this trip so enjoyable. Thank you. "
-Ann D.

"At a time when our life was in a whirlwind with Roy's prostate cancer, your act of kindness, care, and concern has made us feel so much at ease. We appreciate the love you have shown, as we were strangers coming into your business. But you went over and beyond in so many ways. We are humbled by your goodness, expertise, and the many moments you devoted to us. In our lives we sometimes feel we don't deserve it, but you showed your sympathy so we are thankful to God for you. You are an Angel."
-Linda and Ray M.

"Thank you for all you have done for Bill. You helped him tremendously."
-Caroline and William R.

"Thank you so much for helping with the biofeedback treatment. Your patience and encouragement were most helpful. I'm grateful to you for getting my health issues back on track."
-Miriam

"Thank you Vanita for saving my life again. I really appreciate all of your helpful advice and knowledge."
-Claire S.

"Thank you for getting me back to normal. I'm doing really well. I've only had a couple of close calls when I go out. Oh by the way, I told Dr. Desai how much you helped me and she said she'd be sending more patients your way."
-Janet I.

"Words cannot express all that you have done to share your expertise, knowledge, and your encouragement with us as we faced this unknown trial in our lives. We know God places special people in our lives at the exact right time—His time—for a reason. For being there and for all you have done to help us, we are so grateful."
-Gary and Judy M.

"Everything is going fine so far, thank you for your help."
-Rose T.

"Thank you so much for helping me through this challenging period. Your expertise was invaluable, your patience enormous, and we generally enjoyed speaking with you."
-Ron and Bonnie K.

Life after Prostatectomy and Other Urological Surgeries:

10 Weeks from Incontinence to Continence —Vanita's Way

Vanita Gaglani, RPT

Book and book cover design by Jean Boles
http://jeanboles.elance.com

Contents

Acknowledgements

I am grateful to have a very health-care oriented family. My husband, Dr. Mukesh Gaglani, is general practitioner; my daughter, Dr. Anushka Gaglani, is a dentist; and my son, Shiv Gaglani, is a medical student at Johns Hopkins University. He is pursuing his MBA at Harvard this fall. My heart-felt thanks go out to them all. They have encouraged me to write this book so that I can help thousands of people—most importantly, you, dear reader.

A very special thanks to Dr. David M. Albala for writing the Foreword for this book. He is Chief of Urology at Crouse Hospital in Syracuse, New York and is considered a national and international authority in laparoscopic and robotic urological surgery. I appreciate my association with Dr. Albala and his trust in my work with incontinent patients.

Another special thank you to Dr. Boris Havkin, one of the best urologists I have had the fortune to work with. It was Dr. Havkin's forward-looking approach and his innate desire to assist his patients which made him refer his patients to me for physical therapy. That was one of the sparks that jumpstarted my development of a complete protocol for recovering from incontinence post-prostatectomy. Dr. Havkin's patients were among the first to benefit from my program.

Also, special thanks to Dr. Vipul Patel, urologist from Celebration, Florida, who I have had the good fortune to work with. He has performed more than 7000 prostatectomies and in addition has promoted awareness of prostate cancer.

I would also like to thank Dr. Andrew Zabinski, an excellent surgeon and an amazingly good-natured one; Dr. Aimee Tieu, a wonderful urogynecologist who does the best for her patients; Dr. Rader and Dr.

Zipper, both excellent urogynecologists; Dr. Anil Dhople, an excellent radiation oncologist, and Dr. Ravishanker another excellent radiation oncologist.

In addition, I am grateful to the primary care physicians, Dr. Margaret Rank, Dr. Jose Santiago, Dr. Soto Varela, and Dr. Deepti Sadhwani—among others. Also, I would like to express my gratitude to all the other MD's who refer their patients to me.

Last but not least, to my patients, who have been a continual source of inspiration for me. Their confidence in my treatment methods and gratifying improvements—which have often been faster than they, or I, had anticipated—have driven me to work even harder and improve upon my program. Many of the strategies in this book can be traced to experiences I've had with individual patients. It has been a pleasure to work with each of them.

-Vanita Gaglani, RPT

Foreword by David M. Albala, MD

I am honored to have been asked to write the foreword for this book, *Life after Prostatectomy and Other Urological Surgeries: 10 Weeks from Incontinence to Continence—Vanita's Way.*

I feel this book not only will be useful for physicians and other health care providers, but also for patients trying to understand a condition that can be devastating. Currently, it is estimated that a man in the United States has a 1 in 6 (16.6%) lifetime risk of being diagnosed with prostate cancer as a result of clinical symptoms, signs or PSA testing. Prostate cancer accounts for approximately 9% of male cancer deaths and as such, multiple treatments are being recommended for these patients. Urinary continence is a pivotal endpoint with surgical treatment of patients with prostate cancer. In fact, 1 in 7 men may suffer long-lasting urinary incontinence as a result of surgical treatments to the prostate. I challenge readers to deepen their knowledge about urinary incontinence by using this rich resource by Vanita Gaglani.

One of the major barriers to improving incontinence care is a lack of education on the part of health care professionals and patients. Both groups cannot optimally manage a condition that they do not adequately understand. This book is a thorough yet easy to understand summary of urinary incontinence. Here, in one place, is a superb guide to the best practices and tools for managing and treating urinary incontinence. Vanita has gone to great lengths to make urinary incontinence in men after prostate surgery understandable.

She explains the anatomy as well as the role that eating and drinking plays on the bladder. The book contains detailed descriptions of exercises that will be useful for men to regain their lives back. In addition, she describes how a bladder log can serve as an important measure of success. With her program, in ten weeks, most patients will go from wearing numerous pads to no pads at all. This step approach allows patients and their families to have a realistic week-by-week expectation of results without any adverse consequences.

All sections in the book are intended to be short, concise and to the point. The program starts out slowly and gets increasingly more involved. This book will serve as a unique resource for individuals after prostate cancer surgery. It is easy to read and understand as well as being up-to-date. As a registered physical therapy, Vanita Gaglani has been practicing for over 18 years. She understands how incontinence affects lives and how they can be changed in a meaningful way.

I am certain readers will find *Life after Prostatectomy and Other Urological Surgeries: 10 Weeks from Incontinence to Continence—Vanita's Way* informative, practical and clinically relevant.

David M. Albala, MD

Chief of Urology, Crouse Hospital

Syracuse, N.Y.

Preface

Vanita Gaglani has helped hundreds of people gain back control of their bladders and their lives. A registered physical therapist for thirty years, Vanita has practiced for eighteen of those years in Florida. For the past fifteen years, she has specialized in treating urinary incontinence, overactive bladder, and constipation. Vanita's Rehab (phone 321-432-5573) is located in Melbourne, Florida.

During her career in general physical therapy, Vanita learned that many of her patients were also suffering from a silent problem: urinary incontinence—the unintentional loss of urine. Vanita developed a special program for the treatment of incontinence, and some of her first patients were elderly women or women who had recently given birth. Following their successful treatment, these women spread the word of their success, and soon husbands, fathers, brothers and friends also sought help from Vanita.

Many of her patients lead active lives—golfing, biking, traveling, playing with their grandchildren—and many had suffered from the embarrassment of "accidents" or always having to look for a restroom wherever they went. Vanita's has perfected her technique of restoring people's continence, which allows her patients to return to their lives of normalcy within a few weeks after beginning her treatment.

Unique treatment regimen: Vanita's Way

What makes Vanita's Way so unique is that *it works*. There are a lot of programs that rely on some of the same aspects of exercise and nutrition as practiced by her patients; however, although these programs may promote what seems to make sense on the surface, they don't always provide 100% relief from the symptoms of incontinence. Some suggest that patients drink less water to avoid leaking more or to constantly be practicing Kegels to strengthen their pelvic floor muscles faster. Vanita's Way is unique—and it works.

"When it comes to incontinence, I've found three seemingly counterintuitive strategies that are key," she explained. "They are: drink MORE water; wear smaller pads, and do Kegels LESS FREQUENTLY."

Part One:

Introduction

Vanita's Introduction to the
Vanita's Way Program

I have written this book with a lot of encouragement from my patients. Their feedback about what worked and what caused them to leak have been invaluable in the development of this program. A few of them, like Mr. Jim McKinley, were persistent in their efforts to make sure this book was written because they have several friends and relatives around the country who face similar issues of incontinence post prostatectomy, whether it is robotic, laparoscopic, or if they have undergone radiation, or transurethral resection of the prostate (TURP).

Many patients, incontinent following the above surgeries, have found that all the material on the internet and in magazines and books differs widely regarding how many Kegels should be performed, the amount of fluids they should consume, and what kind of activity they should perform post-surgery. When patients have knee, hip, back, shoulder and other surgeries, they are referred to a physical therapist for a structured program to optimize muscle strength and range of motion. Many healthcare providers as well as patients are unaware that *programs do exist to improve pelvic floor muscle strength.*

What makes this book—and the Vanita's Way program—unique is that IT WORKS.

I first started treating male patients when one of them approached me in desperation and asked if I could at least try to help him because I was his last resort. At that time my clientele was females only. He was only sixty-four and was tired of using diapers, urinals and the clamp—which just caused sores on his genitalia. Within a few weeks the gentleman had reduced his usage of about eight diapers daily to none. He was completely continent and rejoined the workforce.

There are a several other programs that rely on some of the same aspects of exercise and nutrition as practiced by my patients. Many of these programs direct patients to decrease their water and fluid intake or perform way too many Kegels. *What differentiates this program is the combination of exercise, behavior and nutrition, which when performed in coordination, promotes continence.*

Being incontinent hurts a man's self-esteem. Women, though aggravated by leaking, are used to wearing pads for multiple years during their menstrual cycles. For men it is frustrating to have a pad pressing on their private parts, a constant reminder of their inability to control leakage.

Whether you picked up this book for a loved one, or you yourself are in need, you can work through the weekly step-by-step plan that has been perfected through continuous feedback from hundreds of patients over the last decade.

The aim of this book is to regain continence through proven, yet conservative measures, including exercise, nutrition, and behavior modification. Just as the knees and hips do post-surgery, any muscle takes a few weeks to strengthen and recover. *Continence can be achieved with persistence and structure and by following the weekly guidelines in this book.*

Chapter One:

Understanding Incontinence in Men (Prostatectomy)

"Before surgery, many men focus on impotence as the major complication of radical prostatectomy. They're wrong. Recovery of urinary control is far more important and—if it happens slowly or doesn't happen at all—casts a far greater shadow on your life. If something's wrong with your ability to urinate, you'll be reminded of it several times a day—or worse, several times an hour—not just a few times a week or month. And frankly, having to change your adult diaper because you just involuntarily urinated in it can dampen— literally—any romantic thoughts that you do have."

-Dr. Patrick Walsh's *Guide to Surviving Prostate Cancer*

Incontinence Myths

You're likely reading this book because you or a loved one is either preparing for surgery for prostate cancer, or has already had an operation. The good news is that the prognosis after prostate cancer is fairly good, especially if the cancer is caught early enough. The bad news is that the surgery may have some side effects that really reduce one's quality of life.

As the quote from Dr. Patrick Walsh makes clear, incontinence is one of the most interruptive side effects experienced after prostate surgery. It's also one of the least discussed and treated side effects, in part due to the following **two myths**:

> *Myth one: Incontinence is a "normal" part of aging.* Given the potential causes of incontinence, many of my patients are older than 40. There is a pervasive rumor that above that age

the occasional leak becomes a normal, and thus, acceptable, part of life. That is completely wrong. I've helped patients in their 80s restore their bladder control to normal and thus, return to active lifestyles.

Myth two: Incontinence only affects women. Urinary incontinence affects both males and females. More than a quarter of men with prostate conditions experience urinary incontinence—about 1 in 5 in the general male population experience it (compared to 1 in 3 in women). (WebMD; http://www.ncbi.nlm.nih.gov/pubmed/17070268),

Given the above myths it often takes months, and in some cases years, before a patient comes to me, by which time he has implemented certain behaviors and habits which take longer to undo. Fortunately, since you are reading this book hopefully you are pre-empting this process or catching it relatively early on.

We'll soon discuss how prostate cancer and surgery actually lead to urinary incontinence, but first we'll take a quick tour of pelvic anatomy so you understand the exercises to come.

Pelvic anatomy

Just as a quick review, urine is filtered out in the kidneys and transported to the bladder where it is stored. The bladder connects to the urethra, which passes through the prostate on its way to the penis and external opening. Incontinence after prostate surgery directly results from damage to the structures adjacent to the bladder that control outflow of urine. These fall into three categories:

1. Physical structures. There are three main structures which play an important role in the return of continence.

a. The internal sphincter at the neck of the bladder. It is here that the maximum damage may occur because the excision at the bladder neck cannot be predetermined and a large area may be involved. It depends on multiple factors, such as encroachment of the prostate, muscle tone of the detrusor muscle, and the muscle tone at the neck of the bladder, since that is composed of smooth muscles.

b. The internal sphincter and the distal prostatic urethra.

c. The Rhabdo sphincter, which is just above the pelvic floor sphincter and at the apex of the prostate. It is the distal urethral external sphincter which determines on how continent you will be. As a result of the surgery the patient remains reliant only on the function of the one remaining external (skeletal muscle or Rhabdo) sphincter.

Perineal Muscles

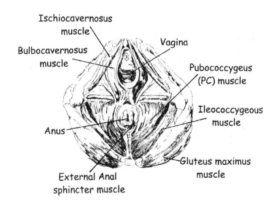

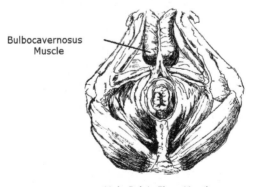

Male Pelvic Floor Muscles

While the use of pads is more acceptable for females, males find it more difficult to get used to pads. Not only is their self-esteem affected, a pad can be uncomfortable for men because of pressure on the scrotum. They also sometimes experience embarrassment from carrying pads or diapers in their pockets, suitcases—or their wife's purse.

2. **Blood vessels.** It's important to get a skilled surgeon, because in some prostate surgeries the blood vessel that supplies the external sphincter may be damaged, leading to damage of the sphincter itself.

3. **Nerves.** Surgeons make every effort to preserve the nerves around the prostate, because damage can result not only in impotence but also in incontinence.

Pelvic floor muscles (PFM)

Think of the pelvic floor muscles as a muscular trampoline at the base of your pelvis. In men, there are two openings through the pelvic floor, for the urethra and anus, while in women there is an additional opening for the vagina.

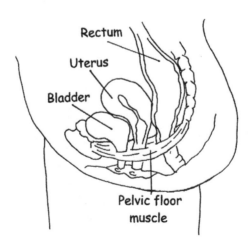

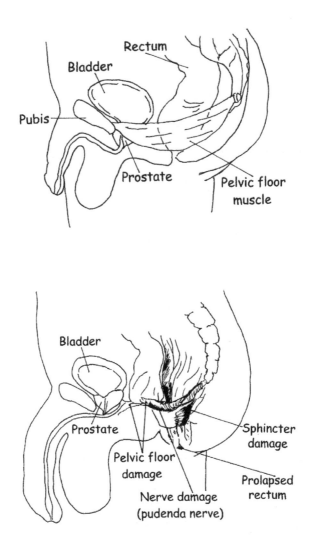

Tightening the pelvic floor muscles elevates the pelvic muscles and constricts the openings mentioned above. Thus, they can be effective tools to prevent the leakage of urine.

The PFM are under voluntary control and, like any muscle, can be strengthened through exercises. Much of this book is devoted to effective exercises that will help you strengthen your own PFM so that you can recover from the potential damage to your pelvic anatomy during surgery.

Vanita's Way

There are literally thousands of self-improvement books that prescribe diet, exercise, and other lifestyle changes—I've read many of them. It's very hard to actually make the prescribed changes because, to be honest, change is difficult. While knowledge from books is helpful, knowledge without action is useless when it comes to seeing progress. So what makes this book different? Enumerated below are the three key reasons that will encourage and assist you in making these changes:

1. First, this book is intended for men who suffer from incontinence especially due to prostate surgery. The strategies have been tailored to fit their needs.

2. Second, incontinence immediately lowers your quality of life and, in many cases, your self-esteem. Golfing and other activities become almost impossible and trips out become a source of potential embarrassment and stress. Thus, my patients, and presumably you or your loved one, are highly motivated to overcome incontinence.

3. Third, I have boiled down the book to essential "Must-Do" and "Take-Home" points so that you have a highly structured and step-by-step program for improvement.

How to receive the greatest benefits from this book

Whether you are picking up this book for a loved one, or you yourself are in need, you can work through the week-by-week plan that has been perfected through continuous feedback from hundreds of my patients over the last decade.

Week 0 describes what you should be doing prior to and immediately after surgery. Advance preparation can make a world of difference when it comes to your recovery, so I strongly urge you to begin following the advice as early as possible. An increasing proportion of my patients are referred to me prior to their surgery because their physicians have seen the excellent results from at least one pre-surgical visit. This empowers my patients with the knowledge of not only what to expect, but what they can do to speed up their recovery post-prostatectomy.

If you missed Week 0, do not fret. The core part of the program begins at Week 1, which is as soon as the catheter has been removed post-surgery, or as soon as you pick up the book after this point—whichever comes first.

The remaining weeks progressively build up your pelvic floor health, so that by the end of the program, you'll be close to normalcy. It is very important to closely follow the regimen. The less you adhere to the program, the more you will leak—it's as simple as that.

The program starts out slowly and gets increasingly more involved. While it will not take much time if you actually calculate it, there are a number of workouts that are cumulatively added, similar to the song "The Twelve Days of Christmas." *I repeat how to do these in each chapter for your convenience*. Consider these a small investment in the short-term so that you can live freely and normally for the rest of your life.

Now, what are the core tenets of the program? As a physical therapist who has trained both in the United States and in India, I strongly believe in the power of lifestyle changes. The aim of this book is to regain continence through proven, yet conservative measures, including exercise, nutrition, and behavior modification. These are generally less expensive than drugs or invasive surgery, and more importantly, have fewer side effects.

27

As a side note, however, it is important to listen to your clinicians and make sure that the changes you are making are in line with your existing exercise, dietary, and medication regimens. I have not had any patients who have had adverse consequences as a result of the program I prescribed, so you can rest easy. However, make sure that any changes you incorporate are gradual and that you regularly monitor how you are feeling throughout the program.

With that background information taken care of, let us dive right into the foundations for restoring your continence, and your life:

- Eating and Drinking Correctly
- Kegels and Other Exercises
- Measuring Success with the Bladder Log

Chapter Two:

Eating and Drinking Correctly

Diet is arguably the most important yet overlooked aspect of regaining your continence. Many patients come to me after unsuccessful attempts at restoring their control, and I ask them about the different regimens they have tried. It always amazes me how simple yet effective options are often missed. Fortunately, you can rest assured that the strategies below have helped hundreds of my patients.

The Importance of Water in Controlling your Bladder

The most important strategy is to drink enough water! This may sound counterintuitive; after all, isn't the problem *too much* urine? No, the problem is a lack of being able to control the release of the urine. The solution is not drinking less; that can lead to dehydration and worsen your incontinence.

There are two main reasons you must drink enough water:

1. Maintaining bladder size

Your bladder is a muscle and can increase or decrease in size, just like your stomach. If you do not drink enough fluids, over time it will shrink. This means that the first sensation to urinate will appear at a lower volume of urine. For example, instead of going to the restroom when you have 150 milliliters (ml—5.0721 US fl. oz.) of urine, you'll feel the urge to go at 50 ml. Shrinkage of the bladder can lead to an urgency to urinate and the need for frequent urination.

To put this in perspective, think of the stomach. A larger stomach can hold more food, which is why some people who want to eat less and lose weight get their stomach stapled so that they feel full with less food consumed. The problem is the reverse with the bladder; you want a bladder that can accommodate more urine without you having to rush off to the bathroom frequently.

Furthermore, if the bladder shrinks in size, it stays in the pelvis and does not expand upwards into the abdomen. This results in it getting pushed by the rectum whenever there is fecal material in the lower intestines. This increased pressure on the bladder leads to liquid leaking.

Also, when you don't drink enough water your fecal material becomes harder, and that can lead to constipation. Constipation is related to incontinence because the more pressure you have in your digestive tract, the more likely it is to push on your bladder and cause you to leak.

2. Maintaining urine balance

Urine has a normal pH of between 5.8 and 7.0. Below 5.5 is highly acidic and causes urgency and frequency. Above 7.5 is very alkaline and is a precursor to bladder infections. Water has a neutral pH, and thus can dilute acidic or basic urine pH levels.

Think of this like the bleach we use for household purposes. 100% bleach will aggravate or even burn your skin; however, we commonly use 10% bleach/90% water as a cleaning solution because it poses less risk. We want our urine to be mostly diluted by water, so that it does not aggravate our urinary system.

Adding some lemon to make water more palatable is acceptable for patients who dislike water alone. For my patients who cannot stand drinking more than a glass of water, milk is a good alternative. Whole, two percent, one percent and skimmed are all fine, although it's recommended to avoid sweetened or flavored varieties.

Here is a brief info on the different types of milk:

1. **Preferred Milk**: Regular, skimmed, 2% and 1%

2. **Soy Milk**: It is the next best alternative for patients who are lactose intolerant. Soy milk is made from dry beans, which are ground after they have been soaked.

The protein value is the same as milk. It is low in carbohydrates. The calorie count is 80~140 Kcal per cup (*A kilocalorie, or Kcal in abbreviated form, is a measurement of the amount of energy in the foods you eat. Low-energy foods have a relatively small amount of kilocalories, while high-energy foods have a lot of kilocalories.*) It is high in phytic acid, isoflavones, and phytoestrogens. It may have been obtained from genetically modified beans.

3. **Coconut milk**: It does not have much protein, has a moderate amount of carbohydrates, about 5 grams of fat and is about 80~90 Kcal per cup.

4. **Almond milk** is obtained by grinding soaked almonds. It is fortified with multiple additives, and is high in carbohydrates.

5. **Hemp Milk** is obtained from the hemp seed. It is high in carbohydrates, fat and sugar, low in protein, and is about 100~140 Kcal per cup.

6. **Rice milk** is obtained from mixing one cup of cooked brown rice and 4 cups of water. Tapioca or carrageenan may be added to it to thicken it. It is low in protein, high in carbohydrates and sugar. It is about 120~130 Kcal per cup.

So how much water should you aim to drink?

Guidelines often recommend 8 glasses of water daily, but rather than measuring out each cup, a better rule of thumb is to drink enough to make sure your urine is pale yellow. Not everyone needs 8 glasses a day, some may need more and some may need less, depending upon your level of activity. For example, if you spend a lot of time outside gardening or golfing, you'll need more water than if you spend much of your time indoors.

Water is an important part of the equation, but also important are the actual substances that you're putting in your body—that is, the food.

The Importance of Food in Controlling your Bladder

Broad considerations for food intake: the good, the needed, and the irritants

- **Irritants**. There are many substances that can irritate your bladder, worsening incontinence. Irritants to avoid include carbonated drinks, tea, coffee, chocolate, citrus fruits, juices, and artificial sweeteners like NutraSweet, Equal, and Splenda. It is much better to consume small portions of brown or pure sugar, or avoid added sugars as much as possible. There are many other positive side effects of following these guidelines in addition to restoring your continence.

- **Diuretics**. It's important to give your urinary system a break by avoiding substances that actively promote trips to the restroom. These include alcohol (beer, wine, and spirits) and caffeine. These substances are also known to cause bladder spasms and irritation.

- **Electrolytes**. It's important to maintain a good balance of electrolytes such as sodium and potassium. These help maintain your pH and are essential in determining how much water your body retains versus urinates. For example, too little sodium and your body may compensate by increasing urination; too much sodium and you can develop high blood pressure, leading to gradual kidney disease and other complications. As with many things in life, it is important to keep a good balance, which often starts with diet.

• **pH**. Another key element of diet during this program to restore your continence is to eat foods that don't shift your urinary pH too much. Recall from above that swings in urine pH can aggravate your urinary system. While the body does most of the heavy lifting in terms of buffering our pH levels, it's still best to balance your intake of acidic and alkaline foods, and avoid eating too much of one class without the either. If you were to do so, though, it's best to be more alkaline than acidic. The following are examples of highly acidic and alkaline substances.

–**Acidic:** carbonated water, energy drinks, club soda, alcohol; cocoa (chocolate) dairy products; artificial sweetener such as Sweet and Low, Equal, NutraSweet, and Stevia; black coffee and tea; sweetened fruit juice; most condiments such as ketchup, mayonnaise, vinegar and salted butter; pickles; all processed food; most grains; cheese; most breads, all citrus and tomatoes.

–**Alkaline:** radish, kale, cabbage, lemons, limes, asparagus, collard greens, artichoke, Brussels sprouts, spinach, broccoli, and onion. (http://blog.totalhomecaresupplies.com/content/wp-content/uploads/2013/03/PH_Spectrum.jpg)

The Hit List—Avoidance is the best policy

Given the above considerations, the following foods are important to *avoid as much as possible*—especially during the program to regain your continence and your life. Of course, this advice should be taken in the context of your other dietary requirements; for example, if you have high blood pressure it's important to continue reducing your salt intake. The three main foods that increase leakage are:

ʾch sugar

2. Too much salt

3. Too many preservatives

- All kinds of artificial or non-sugar sweeteners, such as Sweet and Low, Equal, Splenda, Stevia, and Agave. This includes drinks such as Crystal Light, diet sodas, and Kool-Aid.

- Carbonated beverages, energy drinks, V8

- Flavored milks

- Ice cream

- Cookies

- Salted peanuts, potato chips, salted pretzels

- Pay particular attention to light and fat-free yogurt, fat-free ice cream, and fat-free drinks because they often use artificial sweeteners and coloring to make them palatable.

- Artificial syrups, salad dressings, or sauces

- Canned fruits with too much sugar, preservatives, or salt

- Canned soup

- Microwave dinners

- No more than one to two 8 ounce cups of coffee/day. Make sure you drink at least half a glass of water before and after the coffee.

- Pre-brewed teas such as Arizona and Lipton should be avoided.

- Beer, wine, and spirits

The Safe Foods—Staples for your pantry

The *following foods are safe* and often become staples of my patients:

- All fresh or frozen fruit in limited quantities, including bananas, pears, apples, berries, and grapes. Canned fruit is okay as long as not too much sugar has been added.

- 100% fruit juices (okay from concentrate)—no more than 8-12 oz. a day

- Milk—can be 100%, skimmed, 2% or 1%

- Tomato juices and tomato sauces in reasonable amounts

- All pastas and rice

- Bread—brown is better than white—fresh is better than the ones with long shelf life

- Moderately spicy food such as Thai, Indian, and Mexican

- Fresh or Frozen vegetables. In general, fresh is better than frozen or processed food, which tends to be characterized by having a long shelf live.

My patients who follow the above recommendations find that they not only gain continence back more quickly, but also choose to stick with their newfound healthier diets. Now, before you turn to the next chapter on exercises, how about you take a break to drink a nice glass of water?

Chapter Three:

Kegels and Other Exercises

Introduction: The importance of exercise

As a physical therapist who has been practicing for more than 30 years, I have seen a lot of exercises. I know what works and what does not. And of equal importance, I know what my patients will actually be able to incorporate into their daily routines. The exercises I present in this chapter are the bread-and-butter of my incontinence rehabilitation program. When you get to the week-by-week chapters, you'll see that I include variations on the regimen that are meant to ramp you up from incontinent to fully continent.

I also repeat the descriptions in each chapter since I find that repetition leads to consistency, which leads to success. Plus, it's easier than flipping between pages to remember how to do certain exercises.

Additional benefits of these exercises

Fortunately, none of these exercises requires gym memberships and most can be done in the comfort of your own home. They can also have many side benefits beyond restoring your continence.

For example, building your pelvic floor muscles through Kegels can help you burn calories and lose weight. Kegels are also performed for their sexual health benefits, which my patients tell me are often well received.

Though primarily meant to improve your self-control, the breathing exercises in this book may also help decrease your stress levels, reduce your blood pressure, and increase your mindfulness. I have long been an ardent practitioner of breathing exercises, perhaps stemming from my upbringing in India. It is amazing to see the way in which our American society is now adopting Eastern medical practices such as meditation, yoga, and breathing exercises.

The other exercises I describe at the end of this chapter are meant to strengthen your overall pelvic floor. They also have a number of side benefits, such as burning calories and increasing your flexibility so you feel less sore as you walk around.

Important points to keep in mind before reading on

Do not do more than eight (8) sets of Kegels each day. A set involves 10 repetitions. This is important because I have seen many patients who were advised to do as many Kegels as they were able to, which leads to over-exertion and fatigue, actually causing more leakage.

Within reason, and until you are dry, avoid BLT: Bending, Lifting, or Twisting. Repetitive BLT movements while you are trying to recover your continence post-surgery may negatively influence the coordination and contractility of the pelvic floor muscles and sphincter. In addition, intra-abdominal pressure increases when we bend, lift, or twist, and the pelvic floor muscles, which now act as your sphincter, are not yet strong enough to counteract this.

- Try not to lift anything more than 8-10 pounds in weight. That means not doing heavy housework, including, but not limited to, scrubbing, mopping with a cloth mop, vacuuming with a cleaner that is not self-propelled, cleaning the garage, polishing the car, remodeling the bathroom, and picking weeds. Note that this is **not a permanent** prescription, which your spouse may be happy to know!

• Do not perform abdominal, endurance, and free-weight exercises while recovering this week. The only acceptable form of exercise is walking at a slow pace.

• You can do some BLT, such as putting your shoes and pants on, feeding your pet and taking clothes out of the washer/dryer.

Kegel Exercises

Named after Dr. Arnold Kegel, Kegel exercises involve controlled and progressive contractions of pelvic floor muscles. They are meant to improve muscle tone and strength, thus reducing the potential for leakage. Remember that these muscles, such as the levator ani, help maintain continence by increasing urethral closure and strengthening the anal sphincter.

Unlike the smooth muscle of the bladder wall, these striated muscles are under voluntary control, which allows us to target them for exercise, just like any other muscle you would think of working out.

There are important reasons for doing the Kegel exercises to strengthen the pelvic floor muscle:

1. There is an increase in pelvic floor muscle volume and bulking of the muscle.

2. Pelvic floor muscles (PFM) play a strong part in stabilizing the proximal urethra when it is in the abdomen .

3. Per DeLancy 1988, when the Levator Ani Muscle (PFM) contract, the vesical neck moves anteriorly, thereby compressing it in the precervical arc and as a result the urethra closes.

4. Strong PFM increase blood circulation, balance the muscles, and support the organs.

Pelvic floor muscles

Pelvic floor muscles are composed of two types of fibers:

- Type 1—the slow twitch fibers that make up more than 80 percent of the pelvic floor muscles. We use these muscles to generate a slower, intense contraction.

- Type 2—the fast twitch fibers that comprise the remaining 20 percent. They are responsible for quick, forceful contractions. Inactivity, aging, and nerve damage all contribute to a reduction in these fibers, which comprise enough of the pelvic floor muscles to lead to weakness.

General Guidelines for Kegel Exercises

As with any exercise, it is important to perform Kegels with the correct form. Here are the three broad phases of Kegel exercises:

1. Awareness. Before you can work a muscle out, you must be able to locate it. The following strategy is often suggested to become aware of your pelvic floor muscles: *Imagine that you are at a party and suddenly you feel the urge to pass gas. Focus on preventing the flatulence faux pas by tightening your pelvic floor.*

2. Gaining control. Once you've located your pelvic floor muscles, gain control of them. A patient who worked as a photographer suggested the following strategy, which has since helped my other patients: *Visualize your rectum as a camera shutter. Use your pelvic floor muscles to close (contract) or open (relax) the shutter. It's like taking a picture with your pelvic floor!*

3. Strengthening and toning. After a few sessions step 1 and step 2 will become second nature. Therefore, the majority of the Kegel exercise is performed in this step. I have another analogy for you, and this one is my own: *Imagine that your pelvic floor muscle is an* *elevator. Contract your muscle to bring the elevator up into your abdomen, then release it so it returns to the "ground floor."*

a. The general protocol is to do eight (8) sets a day, every 1-2 hours if possible. Each set consists of 10 repetitions, where at a minimum one repetition is raising the elevator (one second) and lowering it again (one second).

b. This should be done every time you remember it. For example, if you are watching TV and the advertisements come on, or if you are driving and stop at a red light. Obviously, be very careful about paying attention to the road in this last case—the Kegels can wait! Eventually, this will become a habit and help you maintain your continence.

c. Make sure you are breathing! Do not hold your breath while performing Kegels. This can make your head hurt. If your abdominal muscles hurt you are likely over-relying on them and should learn to isolate your pelvic floor muscles by putting one hand on your stomach as you do Kegels.

Specific Guidelines for Kegel Exercises Vanita's Way

With the general guidelines above in mind, the following are specific descriptions of how to do the Kegels in my program:

Quick Kegel

These are the Kegel exercises you will be doing for the first few weeks of the program.

- Sit in a comfortable chair, recliner, or sofa.

- Allow your mind to focus on your pelvic floor muscles.

- Begin squeezing your bottom (rectum) with your muscles. As I said above, one of my patients, a photographer, thought of an analogy that many of my patients find helpful. Think of your rectum like the shutter of a camera. Simply close the shutter with your mind.

• Next, imagine that your closed rectum is an elevator. Quickly raise the elevator up towards your stomach. At this stage we may or may not include a hold for a quick count; for example, a count of five (think "one, two, three, four, five" and NOT "one-Mississippi..."). Now bring it back down. Allow your bottom to relax completely.

• Repeat **at most** 10 times in quick succession. It should take you about 45-60 seconds, which means one second to raise the elevator, five quick-holding counts, and one second to lower it.

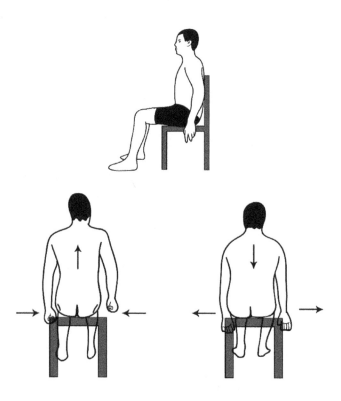

Complete Kegel

The complete Kegel is identical to the quick Kegel with one exception:

- While you are holding the "raised elevator" for a count of three or five, you will simultaneously tighten your penis and scrotum by imagining that you are trying to prevent yourself from urinating. Thus, your entire pelvic region will be tightened for the count.

Frontal Kegel

The frontal Kegel is faster because it only involves tightening the frontal pelvic floor muscles. You can do this by imagining that you are stopping urination mid-stream.

- **Generally you should aim to complete 10 repetitions in around 20 seconds.**

Cough Kegel

- Perform this Kegel while holding in your belly.

- During the quick-holding step, produce an artificial cough. The reason for this is to get your body used to transient increases in intra-abdominal pressure, as coughing or sneezing does. These are times when you're more likely to leak, so we are intentionally simulating it to help you overcome this problem.

After some time diligently performing your Kegels, they will become second nature. **But remember not to overdo it!** A common mistake that patients make is to fatigue their pelvic floor muscles by working them out too much.

It will take about three weeks to begin noticing a reduction in accidents. This can also be recognized by a decrease in the number of pads you have to use, and each time you use the restroom you will have a progressively higher urine output. This is where your bladder log can help you keep track of your progress!

Breathing Exercises

One of the habits I want you to inculcate involves breathing. I instruct my patients to always try to **breathe** on their way to the restroom. Blow small puffs of air through your mouth. Feel the air emerge over your lips. This relaxes your body and takes away your focus from leakage. It also maintains your pelvic floor muscles at an optimum tension; not too relaxed to cause leakage and not too contracted to cause fatigue. Fortunately, breathing exercises can be done multiple times each day without leading to fatigue.

In addition, the following is the key breathing exercise that starts off all other exercises, as described in the next section:

- Breathe in through your nose and out through your mouth.

- Your exhale should be at least twice as long as your inhale; thus, if you breathe in for 3 seconds, breathe out for 6 seconds.

- Make sure you do not become lightheaded when doing these exercises; if you do, you are doing too many.

Additional Exercises

All of these exercises will be added sequentially every week. Do not perform all of them from week one. Remember to follow the exact protocol.

Leg rolls

- Lie down on your back with your legs straight and spread apart by about 12 inches.

- Inhale slowly and roll both legs inward. At the same time gently squeeze your bottom and hold for a quick count of three, five, or seven, depending on the week.

- Now exhale, roll both legs outward, and relax your bottom.

- Repeat the above 10 (or 12, 15, 20 times, depending on the week) to complete the set.

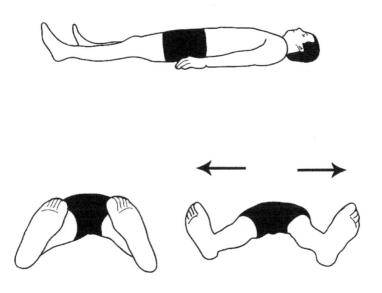

Ball squeeze

A few notes: It's most comfortable to do this exercise on a bed. You will need a soft, rubber ball. I highly recommend the cheap (usually under $2) 9-inch diameter balls at Walmart. Other balls, such as a football or basketball, are too sturdy.

• Lie down on your back with your knees bent and pointed upwards and feet flat on the bed.

• Place the ball between your knees.

• Inhale slowly while squeezing the ball and simultaneously squeezing your bottom (remember the elevator traveling towards your belly) for a quick count of three, five, or seven, depending on the week.

• Release and repeat for a total of 10 (or 12, 15, 20 times, depending on the week) to complete the set.

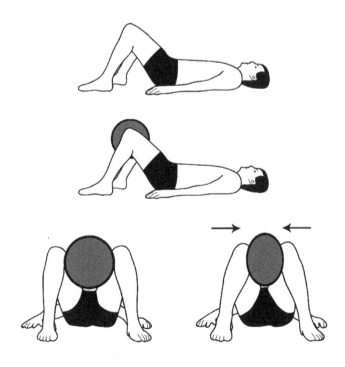

Stretch band abduction

This exercise is basically the opposite of the ball squeeze and instead of adducting your legs you will be *abducting* them (moving them farther apart).

• Lie down on your back with your knees bent and pointed upwards and feet flat on the bed. Your legs can be close together at the starting position.

• Place the stretch band around both thighs, about 3 inches above your knees.

• Slowly move your knees apart about 8-10 inches, against the increasing tension in the band. Hold for a quick count of three, five, or seven, depending on the week.

• Repeat the above 10 (or 12, 15, or 20 times, depending on the week) to complete the set.

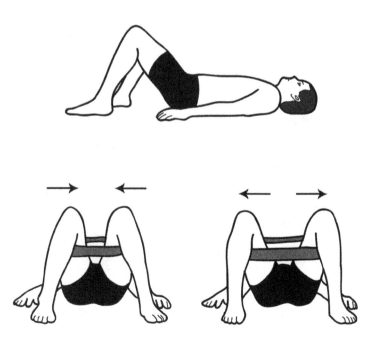

Reverse abdominal

• Lie on your back and bend both of your knees. Place your hands around one of your knees.

• Now lift that leg up so that your thigh is 90 degrees to the surface you're lying on and your knee is perpendicular to your thigh. Then bring the knee to your chest, while your hands gently push back to provide resistance. Hold for a quick count of five.

• Complete five repetitions to finish the set before switching over to the other leg and doing the same. Remember to do two sets each day: morning and evening.

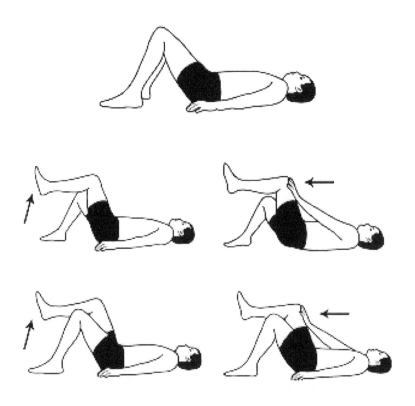

Leg lift

This also works out your abdominals. This exercise and the one above are preferable to crunches because crunches increase the abdominal pressure more significantly, potentially leading to increased leaking.

- Lie on your back with one leg bent and the other straightened on the surface.

- Raise the straight leg up to about 70 degrees. Hold it for a quick count of five, then bring it down.

- Complete five repetitions to finish the set before switching over to the other leg and doing the same. Remember to do two sets each day: morning and evening.

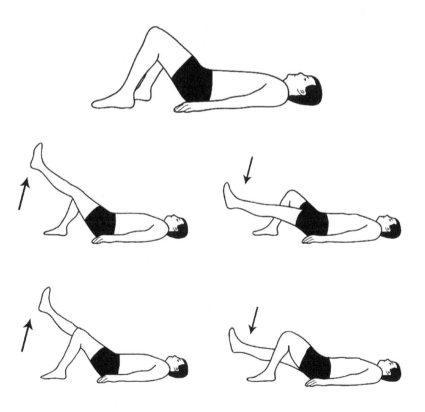

Feet lift

This exercise is similar to those on the previous page.

• Lie flat on your back with both legs bent and your feet flat on the surface.

• Lift **both** feet simultaneously so that your thighs are perpendicular to the surface and your lower legs are parallel to it. Put another way, your thighs would be at a 90-degree angle to your torso and your calves would be at a 90-degree angle to your thighs.

• Hold for a quick count of five, and repeat five times total to complete the set. Do two sets each day: morning and evening.

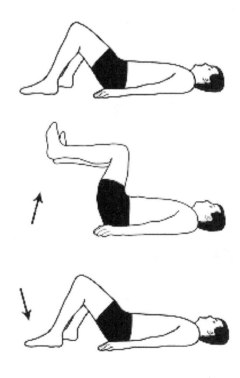

Pillow squeeze

- Lie flat on your back with both legs bent and your feet flat on the surface.

- Place a normal-sized pillow (e.g. width is about six inches) between your knees. Squeeze for five seconds and release.

- Repeat this exercise 10 times to complete a set. As with the others, complete two sets.

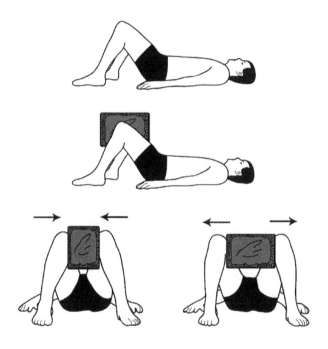

Mini squat

• Stand behind a chair, grasping the top bar firmly. Keep your feet shoulder-width apart.

• Inhale while doing a full Kegel, pulling in your belly, and squatting partway. Do not go all the way down where your thighs are parallel to the ground; instead, do a mini squat.

• Now exhale while standing up and relaxing your pelvic floor muscles.

• Two sets of 10 repetitions each.

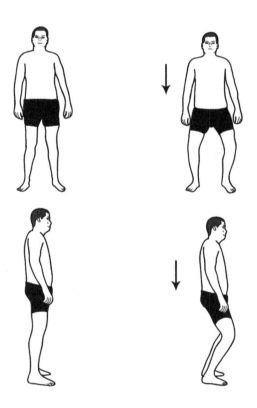

The restroom exercise

If you want to recover even sooner, here's a secret exercise that you can incorporate into your restroom breaks.

- After you're finished on the toilet, sit with your back straight, count to 30 seconds, then lean forward and push like you are releasing gas. Repeat for a total of two times.

- The point of this is to "double-void" and empty the bladder out completely, so there is no residual urine left. This gets your body in the habit of complete emptying, which is important to prevent leakage and accidents after standing up.

There you have them—all of the exercises you need to regain control of your bladder and your life!

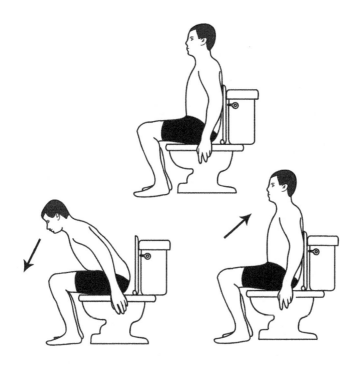

Chapter Four:

Measuring Success with the Bladder Log

Introduction

The famous Irish mathematician, Lord Kelvin, famously stated, "If you cannot measure it, you cannot improve it." This sentiment applies to rocket ships and bladder health alike.

Many people do not know their bodies well enough to notice small, gradual changes, so they become frustrated because they do not see their progress. This is why so many people give up on losing weight and endurance training.

It is also one of the most likely reasons you may give up on this program, which is why I want to introduce the concept—and importance—of logging your results in your "bladder log" at this point in the book. My patients who stick to their bladder logs develop good habits, and they are enthused by the progress they see. This turns the logging process into a positive feedback loop.

Bladder Log

The bladder log is one of the most important tools in our journey to overcome incontinence. Not only does it give you a record of your progress, but it also serves as a reminder to continue with your exercises and nutrition.

Below is the bladder log that I give to all of my patients. Let me take a few minutes to explain what each of the sections represents.

A. Time. We have included 12 rows that each represents a two-hour block of time, beginning at 6 am one day and ending at 6 am the next day. This provides enough resolution for us to identify patterns that may emerge. It's important to keep the log on hand so that you can document as much as you can. For example, if you wake up at 3 am to go to the restroom you'll have it handy to document that entry.

B. Type of Fluid. (W = Water, C = Coffee, T = Tea, J = Juice, M = Milk; 1 cup = 8 oz.) Remember from an earlier chapter that we recommend drinking plenty of water and staying away from caffeinated and acidic beverages. Do your best to document whatever you're drinking. This is often where I spot important, yet easily fixable issues in my patients.

C. Amount Voided. (Short counting: 1, 2, 3…not "one-Mississippi") Anytime you go to the restroom to urinate, get in the habit of steadily counting the duration of the stream. We want the duration to increase, meaning that you are filling up your bladder to larger volumes.

D. Amount of Leakage. (S = small, few drops/dribble; M = medium, wet pad; L = large, change pad) The key on the bladder log describes this fairly clearly. Hopefully, as you go through the program, you'll see more S's and N/A's than L's and M's.

E. Was Urge Present? (1 = mild, first sensation of need to go; 2 = moderate, stronger sensation/start looking for bathroom; 3 = strong, need to go to the bathroom NOW) As with part D, we want to see strong urges (3) being replaced by mild (1) or nonexistent urges.

F. Activity with Leakage. (C = coughing, L = lifting, S = standing, W = walking, SL = sleeping, ST = sitting) There are many reasons for leakage, and this column will help us spot patterns to work on. For example, many C's signify that you leak when you cough, and thus, you may have stress incontinence.

G. Pad/Type. As you go through the program you'll find that I sequentially reduce your pad dependency from heavy (5 dots) to very light (1 dot) and even separate what type you wear based on time of day as well as your routine.

H. Percent Wet. (10% = dollar spot; 50% = 2" x 2"; 100% = soaked) When you do leak, approximately how wet is the pad?

Bladder Log

A	B	C	D	E	F	G	H
Time	Type of Fluid	Amount Voided	Amount Leaked	Was Urge Present?	Activity with Leakage?	Pad/Type	Percent Wet
6 am - 8 am							
8 am - 10 am							
10 am - 12 pm							
12 pm - 2 pm							
2 pm - 4 pm							
4 pm - 6 pm							
6 pm - 8 pm							
8 pm - 10 pm							
10 pm - 12 am							
12 am - 2 am							
2 am - 4 am							
4 am - 6 am							

Download your bladder log

For your convenience we have made the bladder log available at **www.vanitasrehab.com/.** Please download and/or print so that you can fill it out on a daily basis. I give my patients a folder with ample copies of the bladder log, which once filled out provides a record of their progress to show me at our weekly meetings.

Make using the bladder log a habit. Whether that entails setting a daily reminder email to yourself or keeping copies of the log near your bed, in your car, or at your desk at work—do whatever it takes to get tracking.

If you love using your smartphone, there are also a number of apps that may be helpful. I do not have personal experience with these, but it may be worth it to take a look:

- BladderTrackHer (American Urogynecologic Society)
- iP Voiding Diary (Synappz BV)
- Plog (Monsterworks)
- Bladder Pal 2 (Ronald L. Yap, M.D.)
- UroBladderDiary (BillCarithers)

Now what are you waiting for? Get logging!

Part Two:

Continence in Ten Weeks

Chapter Five

Table Outline of the Program

0 – Prepare for a New Lifestyle	
Must-Do-Protocol	• Hydrate • Eat correctly Develop muscle memory
Pads	*Not applicable*
Kegels	Two weeks or more from surgery: • Holding Kegel plus five Kegels in quick succession comprise 1 repetition • 8 sets of 10 repetitions Less than two weeks from surgery: • Complete 10 repetitions of quick Kegels (20 seconds/set) After surgery: No Kegels!
Other Exercises	• Walk, walk, walk. Stay lightly active (within reason) before and after surgery to speed up recovery
Expected Progress	*Not applicable*
Week 1 – Start Slow	
Must-Do-Protocol	• No more than 8 sets of Kegels • Pull in belly often • Relax your bottom
Pads	At Home: • Heavy absorbency pads all day Outside: • Depends or diapers
Kegels	• Complete **up to** 10 repetitions of quick Kegels (20 seconds/set) • Repeat no more than 8 sets
Other Exercises	• Breathe slowly every time you go to restroom to relax your body and maintain pelvic floor muscle tension.
Expected Progress	**Take. It. Slow.** In general patients only start noticing progress around week 3. Give your body time to heal after surgery and as it gets used to this new regimen.

Week 2 – Holding the Count	
Must-Do-Protocol	• No more than 8 sets of Kegels • Pull in belly often • Relax your bottom • Breathe on your way to the restroom
Pads	At Home: • Morning: medium pads • Afternoon: heavy pads Outside: • Depends or diapers
Kegels	• Same as above, except once the elevator is raised hold for a quick count of **three** before releasing (30-45 seconds/set) • Repeat no more than 8 sets
Other Exercises	Two sets of 10 repetitions • Deep breathing • Leg rolls • Ball squeeze
Expected Progress	Some patients report being able to use the same number of heavy pads as diapers, which is an improvement since the heavy pads can only absorb a fraction of fluid that the diapers can. That means they have potentially improved without even realizing it.

Regarding pad usage:

Week 3: Start sitting without a pad for 10 to 15 minutes daily.

Week 4: Start sitting without a pad for 45 minutes to 1 hour.

Week 5: You should have minor leakage in your pad-free time.

Week 6: You should be able to get up and go to the bathroom, kitchen, computer room, etc. without using a pad.

Week 3 –Be Consistent, and Dependent	
Must-Do-Protocol	Same as above
Pads	Introducing pad-free time! At Home: • Morning after exercise: no pads for 10-15 minutes • Medium pads all day Outside: • Heavy pads, avoid Depends or diapers
Kegels	• Same as above, except once the elevator is raised hold for a quick count of **five** before releasing (45-60 seconds/set) • Extra cough Kegel after each set • Repeat no more than 8 sets
Other Exercises	Two sets of 12 repetitions • Deep breathing • Leg rolls • Ball squeeze • Stretch band Hold for a quick count of 3 during each repetition
Expected Progress	By the end of week 3 you should notice a few improvements: - You should have minimal leakage while sleeping, as evidenced by a relatively dry pad when you wake up. - If you do wake up at night to go to the restroom, you should notice that you can reach the toilet without leaking. Once you are there, the duration of your stream should be longer, meaning you have successfully voided. - During the day you should also require less pads. For example, if a patient of mine uses 10 pads on Monday by the following Sunday he may be using 7 pads. Ideally this decrease will be 30-50 percent. Don't forget these are also smaller pads, so it's a double improvement.

Week 4 – Heating Up	
Must-Do-Protocol	Same as above
Pads	At Home: • Morning after exercise: no pads for 30-40 minutes. Holding exercise when you get up. • Medium-to-light pads all day Outside: Medium-to-heavy pads, avoid Depends or diapers.
Kegels	Same as above
Other Exercises	Two sets of 12 repetitions • Breathing • Leg rolls • Ball exercises • Stretch band Two sets of 5 repetitions • Reverse abdominals • Hold for a quick count of 3 during each repetition Add: Restroom exercise
Expected Progress	By the end of week 4 you should be able to get up in the night when you need to use the restroom without leaking. It should be natural like it was prior to surgery. Another sign of progress that you should notice is that you will be barely wet at night (maybe 10%). Assuming that you have no other sleeping difficulties, you should notice that you are sleeping for longer periods of time.

Week 5 – Over the Hump	
Must-Do-Protocol	• No more than 8 sets of Kegels • Pull in belly often • Relax your bottom • Standing relaxation Breathe on your way to the restroom
Pads	At Home: • Morning after exercise: no pads for 1 hour and 15 minutes. Holding exercise when you get up. • Medium-to-light pads all day Outside: • Full transition to medium pads
Kegels	• Same as above, except once the elevator is raised hold for a quick count of **five** while tightening your penis/scrotum before releasing (45-60 seconds/set) • Extra cough Kegel after each set • Repeat no more than 8 sets
Other Exercises	Two sets of 12 repetitions • Breathing • Leg rolls • Ball exercises • Stretch band Two sets of 5 repetitions • Reverse abdominals • Leg lifts • Hold for a quick count of 5 during each repetition Restroom exercise
Expected Progress	By the end of week five you should notice a few significant improvements, such as the ability to: - Sit without a pad for more than two hours. - Sleep without a pad at night and still be dry. - Make it to the bathroom in the morning without leaking, and every hour or so thereafter. Your stream will still be short. - Wear two-dot pads at home, which get about 50% wet, and no longer completely soaked.

Week 6 – Dry at Night	
Must-Do-Protocol	Try to stay without pads for as long as possible. You may stand up and walk to the kitchen, the bathroom, around the house, etc.
Pads	At Home: • Morning after exercise: no pads for 10-15 minutes. Holding exercise when you get up. Afterwards a Rest of day: light pads • Sleep: no pads Outside: • Quick trips (<1 hr.): 1 dot • Long trips: 2 dots. Light pads, avoid Depends or diapers.
Kegels	• Alternating sets of complete and frontal Kegels • Extra cough Kegel after each set
Other Exercises	Two sets of 15 repetitions • Breathing • Leg rolls • Ball exercises • Stretch band Two sets of 5 repetitions • Reverse abdominals • Leg lifts • Feet lifts • Hold for a quick count of 5 during each repetition Restroom exercise
Expected Progress	After week six you should notice the following: - You are almost dry till mid-morning. In the evening after 5 or 6 pm you should also be dry, especially if you decrease your activity. - The afternoon, e.g. 2-4 pm, will be your most leaky period, but we'll decrease that soon enough. - You are using fewer one-dot pads at home, perhaps one every two hours. This equates to about a tablespoon of leakage. Much better!

Week 7 – Dry in the Morning	
Must-Do-Protocol	Perform the following randomly: do a Kegel, tighten the belly at the same time and mimic movements like turning, rolling, picking something, reaching for something. These are the most common movements when leakage occurs and by contracting the belly and performing a Kegel at the same time we preempt the leakage.
Pads	At Home: • Same as above Outside: • Quick trips (<2 hrs): 1 dot • Long trips: 2 dots. Light pads, avoid Depends or diapers.
Kegels	• Complete Kegels for sets 1 and 8; Frontal Kegels for sets 2 through 7 • Extra cough Kegel after each set
Other Exercises	Two sets of 15 repetitions • Breathing • Leg rolls • Ball exercises • Stretch band Two sets of 5 repetitions • Reverse abdominals • Leg lifts • Feet lifts Two sets of 10 repetitions • Pillow squeeze • Hold for a quick count of 5 during each repetition Restroom exercise
Expected Progress	After week 7 you should notice the following signs of progress: - You should be dry in the morning, meaning no pads at all during that time. - During your trips outdoors you should be fine with one-dot pads for short distances and two-dot pads for longer periods of time. If you stay dry, causing the pads to scrunch up and aggravate the scrotum, you may also switch to women's panty liners outside the house for long distances and no pads for short distances. - You should be able to restart your normal activities, such as golf, shopping, and housework.

Week 8 – Getting Back to Normal	
Must-Do-Protocol	Same as above
Pads	At Home: • Morning after exercise: no pads for 10-15 minutes. • Holding exercise when you get up. Afterwards a pantyliner. • Rest of day: 1 dot • Sleep: no pads Outside: • 1 dot for all trips.
Kegels	• Set 1 and 8 are complete Kegels; Sets 2 through 7 are frontal-only – but do these slower: in 30 seconds versus 20 seconds. • Extra cough Kegel after each set
Other Exercises	Two sets of 20 repetitions • Breathing • Leg rolls • Ball exercises • Stretch band Two sets of 10 repetitions • Reverse abdominals • Leg lifts • Feet lifts Two sets of 10 repetitions • Pillow squeeze • Mini squat • Hold for a quick count of 5 during each repetition Restroom exercise
Expected Progress	After week 8 you should be completely pad free inside of the house and require fewer pads during your trips outside of the house (all should be one-dot). You can continue returning to normal activities.

Week 9 – Made It!	
Must-Do-Protocol	Same as above
Pads	At Home: • Morning after exercise: no pads for 10-15 minutes. • Holding exercise when you get up. Afterwards a pantyliner. • Rest of day: 1 dot • Sleep: no pads Outside: • 1 dot for all trips.
Kegels	• Set 1 and 8 are complete Kegels; Sets 2 through 7 are frontal-only – but do these slower: in 30 seconds versus 20 seconds. • Extra cough Kegel after each set
Other Exercises	Same as above
Expected Progress	At this point if all has gone well you should be back to normal! Here's what my patients report at the end of the program: - Normal sensation to urinate, with a good stream. - Dry all day. - Using thin panty liners during exercise and longer trips outside of the house, just in case.

Week 10 – Back to Normal

Chapter Six

Week Zero—Prepare for a New Lifestyle

Introduction

If you are reading this book before your prostate procedure, then this chapter will offer helpful material that can speed up your recovery process so that you regain continence sooner.

An aside: Though I've called this chapter week zero, it may not actually be seven days long. If you pick this book up a month before your operation, then that whole month is week 0. "Week 0" includes any time before Week 1 begins, which is when your catheter is removed.

Fortunately, surgery has become so advanced that you should be able to resume your daily schedule within a few days.

The urologists I've met who perform radical prostatectomies really know their fields and are able to achieve great outcomes. Many other urologists use advanced robotics like the Da Vinci Surgical Robot that, if used by excellent hands, allow them to decrease the overall loss of blood and length of the hospital stay. Still others use techniques such as high intensity focused ultrasound (HIFU) which destroys tissue through heating.

Though outcomes are improving, these procedures still target your pelvic area, which is a small amount of real estate for a lot of very important anatomy.

Regardless of which type of procedure you will undergo there are ways to prepare your body for the upcoming operation. Here is what you can do before and immediately after surgery to improve your chances for a speedy recovery.

Before surgery

You've probably realized from previous chapters that there are a few really important changes that you'll be making to regain your continence and lifestyle post-surgery. So, as Thomas Jefferson famously said, "Never put off till tomorrow what you can do today." If you start getting in the habit of drinking plenty of water, eating the right foods, and performing Kegel exercises, it'll be that much easier for you to recover, since your body will already be used to these changes.

1. Hydrate

In addition to all of the other benefits that come with drinking enough water, it will help expand your bladder and dilute your urine so that your bladder is less irritated.

Remember the key rule is to drink enough so that your urine is pale yellow or clear.

Caveat: Be careful not to go overboard, because too much water can be harmful. It could dilute your sodium and potassium levels, which are very important elements for the proper functioning of your muscles and body.

2. Eat correctly

Recall from an earlier chapter that it is important to avoid irritants and diuretics while regaining your continence. You'll be singularly focused on recovering from your surgery so it's better to start making these changes as early as possible so you do not find yourself having to go "cold turkey." For example, you can gradually wean yourself off of artificial sweeteners and reduce your daily alcohol intake, if any.

3. Muscle memory

Kegels and other exercises will be essential to your recovery. Fortunately, you can develop muscle memory for how to do these correctly. It is a wise choice to get a head start and begin performing these prior to your surgery. Not only will you know how to do them properly when you truly need them, you will also be developing strength in your pelvic floor muscles that can help you recover more quickly.

If your surgery is two weeks or more away, this is the recommended protocol for strengthening your pelvic floor with Kegel exercises:

One (1) repetition consists of the following:

- Hold one Kegel for a count of five,

- Then do five Kegels in quick succession, within 10 seconds (contract in one second, release in another second)

- You will do eight (8) sets of 10 repetitions each. That means 80 repetitions, which means 80 Kegels held for a count of five and 400 Kegels in quick succession.

That sounds like quite a bit, but it should take only 20 minutes or so throughout the whole day. You should spread out the 8 sets, at a minimum spacing of 1 hour. Fortunately, you can do these anywhere you are sitting; for example, while driving, watching TV, or working. The investment in your health now will go a long way and quicken your recovery post-surgery.

If your surgery is less than two weeks away, you can do the above protocol each day **without the holding Kegel**, just 10 Kegels in quick succession. The reason for this is that you do not want to over-fatigue your pelvic floor right before surgery.

4. Bladder log

Though most people only begin their bladder logs after surgery, there is a benefit to starting earlier. It is a good idea to have a baseline measure of your health, especially before any interventions such as prostate surgery. For example, if you had to go to the restroom 5 times each day before surgery and had no leakages, you would know that that's your healthy normal. If your restroom breaks increase to 10 times a day, and you're having 3 leaks on average, then you know exactly how much you have to improve to get back to normal. It requires some time and diligence to track this, but it will be well worth it on your road to recovery.

5. Immediately after surgery

Congratulations! The worst is hopefully behind you and you can begin your journey back to normal life.

I've treated more than a thousand patients for incontinence and the ones who recover the fastest are most always the ones with the most positive attitudes. Do not underestimate how important your mindset will be to your recovery! Now that you're finished with your surgery, this is the beginning of the end of your pelvic floor problems.

So what should you be doing immediately after surgery until your catheter is removed? Many of my patients feel surprisingly well right after surgery and want to "run before they can walk." While you should keep your healthy hydration and eating habits, you should **not** be doing Kegels.

Let me repeat that: **do not do Kegels right after surgery**.

The pelvic floor muscles can get easily fatigued so they will not be able to contract to the maximum potential. You've just had a surgery and even though you feel fine, the individual muscles have undergone major trauma. You need to allow for healing to occur, because otherwise, you'll overwork them and delay your recovery. Give yourself a break—there'll be plenty of Kegels later! And you'll still have your catheter, so it won't be necessary to stop your flow through Kegels.

One interesting note is that prostate surgery is different from other types of surgery in that the incisions are generally smaller and lead to less post-surgical pain. Thus, patients can overdo exercises right after prostate surgery as opposed to, say, knee or shoulder surgery, where the pain limits how much exercise they are able to do.

However, it is still important to stay relatively active. The best thing you can do for your body is to walk, walk, walk. Focus on healing your overall body and being able to get out of the bed, but be responsible about it, and do not overexert yourself. Do not worry about any other exercises for the time being.

Chapter Seven

Week One—Start Slow

Introduction

Now that your catheter has been removed, we're ready to begin the ten-week program to help you regain your continence and your life. We'll be starting slowly with week one.

The first few weeks may be frustrating because you'll be experiencing the symptoms of incontinence and slowly seeing progress. Like anything worth doing, it will be important to stay the course and persevere. Know that thousands of people before you have regained bladder control and thousands of people after you will do so as well. What follows is a tried-and-true method, so rest assured that you will recover. Remember that you must keep a positive mental attitude, as that will help speed up your recovery.

I will be repeating the most important points in each chapter to make sure they are truly driven home. Exercises require proper form, and diet should be closely followed to see the best results. These should be performed each day of the week for best results.

There is a constant repetition to pay attention to be sure that you are not clenching your bottom, because it is natural that when one feels leakage that we try to stop it by "clenching." It becomes a habit and the repetition to relax your bottom breaks that habit.

Must-Follow Advice

Exercise and muscles

- **At most** do eight (8) sets of Kegels each day.

  –DO NOT DO MORE. Doing more will fatigue your pelvic floor muscles. Pelvic floor muscles become taut, and though weak, are able to tighten around the bladder neck, which then will not be able to contract, leading to you leaking more.

- Remember to **pull in your belly**.

The reason we pull in the abdomen (belly) is that the intra-abdominal pressure decreases. Also, if an ultrasound of the bladder is done when we pull in the belly, we are able to observe the bladder neck becoming slender, and therefore, the pelvic floor muscles—though weak—are able to tighten around the neck.

  –Before standing up. Once you are up, let your belly relax gently, but so you do not leak, do not let go completely.

  –Before sitting down. Once you are seated, relax gently.

  –Before bending down. For example, to wipe your feet after a shower, pick something up from the floor, or put your pants or shoes on.

- When sitting make sure your **bottom is relaxed**.

  –If you sit with your bottom squeezed tightly, you will eventually feel pain in your rectal and genital areas. This will lead to increased leakage or the constant urge to urinate with no stream, again due to muscle fatigue.

–This is one reason deep breathing is such an important exercise. Breathe in through your lips, then as you breathe out, relax your bottom.

Pad Protocol

After having seen hundreds of patients, I've developed my own unique protocol when it comes to using pads. These choices will affect your physical and psychological comfort and the speed at which you recover. Some decisions may seem counterintuitive, such as wearing thinner or smaller pads, but they have worked for most of my patients, and I am confident they will work for you. I divide the pad protocol into "Home" use and "Outside" use. But first, some general notes:

–Make sure that the pads are "Ultrathin" so they will fit comfortably in your underwear.

–To wear, remove the sticky tape from under the pad and place inside of your Jockey underwear. Make sure that the underwear is not too tight when you put it on, because the resulting discomfort may cause you to leak more.

–You will likely be changing your protective pads and Depends multiple times each day. Change them when they are soaked (generally 80% or more saturated) for consistency sake, and remember to keep track of how many you're using in the bladder log.

–Each week we will reduce your dependence by decreasing the thickness of the protection you use. For example, if you start with diapers then the next week we'll aim to replace them with 5-dot pads, and then next week to 4-dot pads, and so forth until you are pad-free.

–Note: if your pad is too narrow and doesn't cover the base of your underwear, feel free to double up (or 1.5 x) on them. You may go through them faster, but the eventual goal is to get you to be pad-free, so you'll be saving in the long run—not to mention improving your quality of life—by doubling down and sticking to the regimen.

• Home Pad Use

–Begin using heavy absorbency pads instead of pull-ups. These can usually be identified by the words "Heavy Absorbency" and five dots indicating the heaviest usage.

–The brand does not matter as much, and there are many options including CVS, Walgreens, TENA, and Depends. You may even pick up brands that are usually meant for women, such as Poise and Carefree. Do not be ashamed—pads are simply temporary tools on your road to recovery! Much more embarrassing to you would be living the rest of your life with leakage.

–Make sure that the pads are "Ultrathin" so they will fit comfortably in your underwear. Ultrathin pads do not put pressure on your genital area, which is good for mitigating the risk of leaking. Ultrathin pads, though thin, can absorb heavy amounts of urine.

–To wear, remove the sticky tape from under the pad and place inside of your Jockey underwear. Make sure that the underwear is not too tight when you put it on, because the resulting discomfort may cause you to leak more.

• Outside Pad Use

–Outside of the house you can continue wearing Depends or diapers until you become more confident.

Exercise Protocol

- Important Points

    −Do not do more than eight (8) sets of Kegels each day. A set involves 10 repetitions.

    −Within reason, and until you are dry, avoid BLT: bending, lifting, or twisting. Repetitive BLT movements while you are trying to recover your continence post-surgery may negatively influence the coordination and contractility of the pelvic floor muscles and sphincter. In addition, intra-abdominal pressure increases when we bend, lift, or twist, and the pelvic floor muscles—which are acting as a sphincter and valve—are not yet strong enough to counteract this.

    −Try not to lift anything more than 8-10 pounds in weight. That means laying off heavy housework, including but not limited to scrubbing, mopping with a cloth mop, vacuuming with a cleaner that is not self-propelled, cleaning the garage, polishing the car, remodeling the bathroom, and picking weeds. Note that this is **not a permanent** prescription, which your spouse may be happy to know!

    −Do not perform abdominal, endurance, and free weight exercises while recovering this week. The only acceptable form of exercise is walking at a slow pace.

    -Crunches are a no no!

    −You can do some BLT, such as putting your shoes and pants on, feeding your pet, and taking clothes out of the washer/dryer.

• Kegels

Note that the Kegel protocol changes slightly each week, so it will be important for you to follow the specific steps below while keeping in mind the general form of the exercises as described in an earlier chapter.

–The first step before performing your Kegels is to update your bladder log. Remember that this should become a daily habit so that you keep track of your progress over time.

–Next get into position and practice one Kegel:

1. Sit in a comfortable chair, recliner, or sofa

2. Allow your mind to focus on your pelvic floor muscles.

3. Begin squeezing your bottom with your muscles. One of my patients, a photographer, thought of an analogy that many of my patients find helpful. Think of your rectum like the shutter of a camera. Simply close the shutter with your mind.

4. Next imagine that your closed rectum is an elevator (another analogy). Quickly raise the elevator up towards your stomach, then bring it back down.

5. Allow your bottom to relax completely.

6. Repeat **at most** 10 times in quick succession. It should take you about 20 seconds, which means one second to raise the elevator and one second to lower it.

–Complete **up to** 8 sets of these Kegels each day this week.

• Breathing and Other Exercises

This week involves one simple breathing exercise, which you should aim to do whenever you feel the urge to go to the restroom.

On your way to the restroom begin blowing small puffs of air through your mouth. Feel the air emerge over your lips. This relaxes your body and takes away your focus from leakage. It also maintains your pelvic floor muscles at an optimum tension—not too relaxed to cause leakage and not too contracted to cause fatigue.

Expected Progress

Take It Slow. In general patients only start noticing progress around **WEEK 3**. Give your body time to heal after surgery and as it gets used to this new regimen.

• Take Home Points

I want to end this chapter in the same way that it began: with important points that deserve repetition because they are crucial to your recovery. Let us begin:

–Do not do Kegel exercises constantly; in fact, do not do more than 8 sets of 10 repetitions each day. Remember that the pelvic floor muscles are small, like the muscles of the hand or face, and thus, they fatigue quickly. When they are fatigued they cannot contract tightly, and when they cannot contract you leak more. **The more exercise you do past a certain point, the more you will leak!** This sounds opposite to what society teaches us: "No pain no gain."

–When you are sitting make sure that you relax your rectum and perineal areas. My patients who worry about leaking often sit with them clenched, and thus, fatigue their pelvic floor muscles, leading to more leaking. The worry about leaking becomes a self-fulfilling prophecy!

–Do not try to stop the leakage right away. No matter what you do, there will be at least some dribbling. It will stop. Give it time. It is a muscle. It takes at least 6-8 weeks to notice any changes after exercising other muscles, such as your abdominals or biceps, so remember that the same applies to your pelvic floor muscles. These muscles and the bladder will not strengthen and coordinate in a week!

That concludes the first week on your journey back to normalcy. Celebrate your accomplishments thus far and stick with it!

Chapter Eight

Week Two—Holding the Count

Introduction

Welcome to the second week! I hope the first week went smoothly enough for you. Remember that the first few weeks may be frustrating because you'll be experiencing the symptoms of incontinence and slowly seeing progress. Stay the course and it'll be worth it.

While there are a few changes, many of the strategies in week 2 are repeated to get you into a consistent regimen. As former British Prime Minister Benjamin Disraeli once said, "The secret of success is consistency of purpose." I would make a corollary to that: "The secret of regaining control of your bladder and life is consistency of action."

I will be repeating the most important points in each chapter to make sure they are truly driven home. Exercises require proper form and diet should be closely followed to see the best results. These should be performed each day of the week for best results.

Must-Follow Advice

Exercise and muscles

- **At most** do eight (8) sets of Kegels each day.

  –DO NOT DO MORE. Doing more will fatigue your pelvic floor muscles, which then will not be able to contract leading to you leaking more.

• Remember to **pull in your belly**.

The reason we pull in the abdomen (belly) is that the intra-abdominal pressure decreases. Also, if an ultrasound of the bladder is done when we pull in the belly, we are able to observe the bladder neck becoming slender, and therefore, the pelvic floor muscles—though weak—are able to tighten around the neck.

–Before standing up. Once you stand up, let your abdomen (belly) relax gently, but so that you do not leak too much, do not let go completely. You may feel a dribble, which is perfectly normal at this stage. If you forget to pull in your belly before standing up, sit back down and immediately stand up again, this time with the correct form.

The reason for pulling in your belly is that it stabilizes the bladder.

–Before sitting down. Once you are seated, relax gently.

–Before bending down. For example, to wipe your feet after a shower, pick something up from the floor, or put your shoes on.

• When sitting make sure your **bottom is relaxed**.

–If you sit with your bottom squeezed tightly, you will eventually feel pain in your rectal and genital areas. This will lead to increased leakage, again due to muscle fatigue.

–This is one reason deep breathing is such an important exercise. Breathe in through your lips, then as you breathe out, relax your bottom.

• **Breathe** on your way to the restroom.

–On your way to the restroom, blow small puffs of air through your mouth. Feel the air emerge over your lips. This relaxes your body and takes away your focus from leakage. It also maintains your pelvic floor muscles at an optimum tension— not too relaxed to cause leakage and not too contracted to cause fatigue.

Pad Protocol

After having seen hundreds of patients, I've developed my own unique protocol when it comes to using pads. These choices will affect your physical and psychological comfort and the speed at which you recover. Some decisions may seem counterintuitive, such as wearing thinner or smaller pads, but they have worked for most of my patients and I am confident they will work for you. I divide the pad protocol into "Home" use and "Outside" use. But first, some general notes:

–Make sure that the pads are "Ultrathin" so they will fit comfortably in your underwear.

–To wear, remove the sticky tape from under the pad and place inside of your Jockey underwear. Make sure that the underwear is not too tight when you put it on because the resulting discomfort may cause you to leak more.

–You will likely be changing your protective pads and Depends multiple times each day. Change them when they are soaked (generally 80% or more saturated) for consistency sake, and remember to keep track of how many you're using in the bladder log.

–Note: if your pad is too narrow and doesn't cover the base of your underwear, feel free to double up on them. You may go through them faster, but the eventual goal is to get you to be pad-free so you'll be saving in the long run—not to mention improving your quality of life—by doubling down and sticking to the regimen.

• Home Pad Use

This week at home we'll begin drawing a distinction between morning pad use and pad use throughout the rest of the day. In the morning there is generally less leakage, but as the day progresses a combination of fatigue and gravity weaken the pelvic floor, so there is more leakage.

With this in mind, in the morning (up until 11 am or noon) you can begin using medium absorbency pads.

–These can usually be identified by the words "Medium Absorbency" and three dots. A common brand that my patients use is TENA Twist, though as mentioned above you may have to double up to cover your entire base.

–For 2-3 days you may be frustrated by having to go through your pads more often, but after that you should see a decrease.

–For the rest of the day you can switch back to heavy absorbency (5 dot) pads.

• Outside Pad Use

–Outside of the house you can continue wearing Depends or diapers until you become more confident.

Exercise Protocol

• Important Points:

–Do not do more than eight (8) sets of Kegels each day. A set involves 10 repetitions.

−Within reason and until you are dry avoid BLT: bending, lifting, or twisting. Repetitive BLT movements while you are trying to recover your continence post-surgery may negatively influence the coordination and contractility of the pelvic floor muscles and sphincter. In addition, intra-abdominal pressure increases when we bend, lift, or twist and the pelvic floor muscles are not yet strong enough to counteract this.

−Try not to lift anything more than 8-10 pounds in weight. That means laying off heavy housework, including but not limited to scrubbing, mopping with a cloth mop, vacuuming with a cleaner that is not self-propelled, cleaning the garage, polishing the car, remodeling the bathroom, and picking weeds. Note that this is **not a permanent** prescription, which your spouse may be happy to know!

−Do not perform abdominal, endurance, and free weight exercises while recovering this week. The only acceptable form of exercise is walking at a slow pace.

−You can do some BLT such as putting your shoes and pants on, feeding your pet, and taking clothes out of the washer/dryer.

• Kegels

Note that the Kegel protocol changes slightly each week so it will be important for you to follow the specific steps below while keeping in mind the general form of the exercises as described in an earlier chapter.

−The first step before performing your Kegels is to update your bladder log. Remember that this should become a daily habit so that you keep track of your progress over time.

–Next get into position and practice one Kegel:

1. Sit in a comfortable chair, recliner, or sofa

2. Allow your mind to focus on your pelvic floor muscles.

3. Begin squeezing your bottom with your muscles. One of my patients, a photographer, thought of an analogy that many of my patients find helpful. Think of your rectum like the shutter of a camera. Simply close the shutter with your mind.

4. Next imagine that your closed rectum is an elevator (another analogy). Quickly raise the elevator up towards your stomach.

5. Hold for a quick count of three (think "one, two, three," and NOT "one-Mississippi…"). Now bring it back down.

6. Allow your bottom to relax completely.

7. Repeat **at most** 10 times in quick succession. It should take you about 30-45 seconds, which means one second to raise the elevator, three quick-holding counts, and one second to lower it.

• Breathing and Other Exercises

This week you will be doing two sets of the following exercises, once in the morning and once in the evening. Each set should be 10 repetitions.

–First begin with a set of deep breathing exercises:

1. Breathe in through your nose and out through your mouth.

2. Your exhale should be at least twice as long as your inhale; thus, if you breathe in for 3 seconds, breathe out for 6 seconds.

3. Repeat the above 10 times total to complete the set.

Make sure you do not become lightheaded when doing these exercises; if you do, you are doing too many.

–Next move on to the set of leg rolls:

1. Lie down on your back with your legs straight and spread apart by about 12 inches.

2. Inhale slowly and roll both legs inward. At the same time gently squeeze your bottom and hold for a quick count of 3.

3. Now exhale, roll both legs outward, and relax your bottom.

4. Repeat the above 10 times total to complete the set.

–The final exercise is the ball squeeze.

A few notes: It's most comfortable to do this exercise on a bed. You will need a soft, rubber ball. I highly recommend the cheap (usually under $2) 9-inch diameter balls at Walmart. Other balls, such as a football or basketball, are too sturdy.

1. Lie down on your back with your knees bent and pointed upwards and feet flat on the bed.

2. Place the ball between your knees.

3. Inhale slowly while squeezing the ball and simultan-eously squeezing your bottom (remember the elevator traveling towards your belly) for a quick count of three.

4. Release and repeat for a total of 10 times to complete the set.

Expected Progress

Remember the theme of week one? Take—It—Slow. In general patients only start noticing progress around week three. Channel your inner Benjamin Disraeli and be consistent to reach success.

That being said, some patients do report being able to use the same number of heavy pads as diapers, which is an improvement, since the heavy pads can only absorb a fraction of fluid that the diapers can. That means they have potentially improved without even realizing it.

• Take Home Points

I want to end this chapter in the same way that it began: with important points that deserve repetition because they are crucial to your recovery. Let us begin:

–Do not do Kegel exercises constantly; in fact, do not do more than 8 sets of 10 repetitions each day. Remember that the pelvic floor muscles are small, like the muscles of the hand or face, and thus, they fatigue quickly. When they are fatigued they cannot contract tightly, and when they cannot contract you leak more. **The more exercise you do past a certain point, the more you will leak!** This sounds opposite to what society teaches us: "No pain no gain."

–When you are sitting or walking make sure that you relax your rectum and perineal areas. My patients who worry about leaking often sit with them clenched, and thus, fatigue their pelvic floor muscles, leading to more leaking. The worry about leaking becomes a self-fulfilling prophecy!

–Do not try to stop the leakage right away; however, feel free to maintain a small amount of tension in your pelvic floor muscles. No matter what you do there will be at least some dribbling. It will stop. Give it time. It is a muscle. It takes at least 6-8 weeks to notice any changes after exercising other muscles, such as your abdominals or biceps, so remember that the same applies to your pelvic floor muscles. These muscles and the bladder will not strengthen and coordinate in a week!

That concludes the second week on your journey back to normalcy. Celebrate your accomplishments thus far and stick with it!

Chapter Nine

Week Three—Be Consistent, Not Dependent

Introduction

Welcome to week three! We make some really important changes this week so pay close attention as you read through this chapter.

I will continue repeating the most important points in each chapter to make sure they are truly driven home. Exercises require proper form, and diet should be closely followed to see the best results. These should be performed each day of the week for best results.

Must-Follow Advice

Exercise and Muscles

- **At most** do eight (8) sets of Kegels each day.

    –DO NOT DO MORE. Doing more will fatigue your pelvic floor muscles, which then will not be able to contract leading to you leaking more.

- Remember to **pull in your belly**.

The reason we pull in the abdomen (belly) is that the intra-abdominal pressure decreases. Also, if an ultrasound of the bladder is done when we pull in the belly, we are able to observe the bladder neck becoming slender, and therefore, the pelvic floor muscles—though weak—are able to tighten around the neck.

–Before standing up. Once you are up, let your belly relax gently, but do not let go completely so you do not leak too much. You may feel a dribble, which is perfectly normal at this stage. If you forget to pull in your belly before standing up, sit back down and immediately stand up again, this time with the correct form.

–Before sitting down. Once you are seated, relax gently.

–Before bending down. For example, to wipe your feet after a shower, pick something up from the floor, or put your shoes on.

• When sitting make sure your **bottom is relaxed**.

–If you sit with your bottom squeezed tightly, you will eventually feel pain in your rectal and genital areas. This will lead to increased leakage, again due to muscle fatigue.

–This is one reason deep breathing is such an important exercise. Breathe in through your lips, then as you breathe out, relax your bottom.

• **Breathe** on your way to the restroom.

–On your way to the restroom, blow small puffs of air through your mouth. Feel the air emerge over your lips. This relaxes your body and takes away your focus from leakage. It also maintains your pelvic floor muscles at an optimum tension—not too relaxed to cause leakage and not too contracted to cause fatigue.

• Important Addition to Protocol: Pad-Free Time

This week I introduce an effective strategy that helps my patients get dry faster.

After you perform your first set of morning exercises, remove your pad or other form of leakage protection. Then, while you are sitting down as per your normal routine—for example, eating breakfast, working on your computer or watching TV—do the following:

> 1. Place a plastic bag, such as a garbage bag, on your seat and cover it with a hand towel or small square disposable mattress pad if you would prefer.

> 2. Sit down wearing only your jockey shorts or underwear. These will gradually become soaked, often within 10 minutes, but do not be alarmed. The reason this happens is that you have become used to the protection of the pad, and your mind does not notice or care as much about a damp pad but certainly feels the effect of wet underwear.

>> a. An analogy would be getting in the habit of lifting a full bucket of water each day until your body learns to expect the weight of the full bucket. Then one day the bucket is only half-full but you lift it with the usual amount of force, surprising you when the water spills.

–Once your underwear is wet you can change it and resume using pads the rest of the day.

The reason this exercise is performed in the morning is because you have just slept overnight without using your pelvic floor muscles (PFM), and by lying down there has been relatively little weight on your PFM, your bladder, and your rectum. That means your PFM should be strongest in the morning.

–You will most likely be frustrated when you do this the first few times. The first time you sit down without a pad your underwear may be soaked within 10 minutes. The next time it may be 15 or 20 minutes. If you keep at it, you'll soon be dry for an hour or more.

–The purpose of this exercise is to get your mind and body used to returning to a pad-free lifestyle. Consistency is an important part of success, but dependency needs to be avoided.

Pad Protocol

–Use "Ultrathin" pads (heavy, medium or thin) so they will fit comfortably in your underwear.

–To wear, remove the sticky tape from under the pad and place inside of your Jockey underwear. Make sure that the underwear is not too tight when you put it on because the resulting discomfort may cause you to leak more.

–You will likely be changing your protective pads and Depends multiple times each day. Change them when they are soaked (generally 80% or more saturated) for consistency sake, and remember to keep track of how many you're using in the bladder log.

–Note: if your pad is too narrow and doesn't cover the base of your underwear, feel free to double up on them. You may go through them faster, but the eventual goal is to get you to be pad-free so you'll be saving in the long run—not to mention improving your quality of life—by doubling down and sticking to the regimen.

• Home Pad Use

The distinction between morning and evening pad use from week two does not apply to week three. Now when you're home you should be using medium absorbency pads all day long.

–These can usually be identified by the words "Medium Absorbency" and three dots. A common brand that my patients use is TENA Twist, though as mentioned above you may have to double up to cover your entire base.

–Initially you may be frustrated by having to go through your pads more often, but after that you should see a decrease.

• Outside Pad Use

–Outside of the house you should make the transition this week to heavy absorbency pads (5 dots), and forego the Depends and diapers. Again, this may be frustrating initially, but we are trying to avoid making your body dependent on, well, Depends.

–You can take extra pads with you in your bag or pocket.

–Feel free to check the pad as often as needed by taking restroom breaks, as frequently as each hour if you need to.

Exercise Protocol

• Important Points:

–Do not do more than eight (8) sets of Kegels each day. A set involves 10 repetitions.

–Within reason and until you are dry avoid BLT: bending, lifting, or twisting. Repetitive BLT movements while you are trying to recover your continence post-surgery may negatively influence the coordination and contractility of the pelvic floor muscles and sphincter. In addition, intra-abdominal pressure increases when we bend, lift, or twist and the pelvic floor muscles are not yet strong enough to counteract this.

−Try not to lift anything more than 8-10 pounds in weight. That means laying off heavy housework, including but not limited to scrubbing, mopping with a cloth mop, vacuuming with a cleaner that is not self-propelled, cleaning the garage, polishing the car, remodeling the bathroom, and picking weeds. Note that this is **not a permanent** prescription, which your spouse may be happy to know!

−Do not perform abdominal, endurance, and free weight exercises while recovering this week. The only acceptable form of exercise is walking at a slow pace.

−You can do some BLT such as putting your shoes and pants on, feeding your pet, and taking clothes out of the washer/dryer.

• Kegels

Note that the Kegel protocol changes slightly each week, so it will be important for you to follow the specific steps below while keeping in mind the general form of the exercises as described in an earlier chapter.

−The first step before performing your Kegels is to update your bladder log. Remember that this should become a daily habit so that you keep track of your progress over time.

−Next get into position and practice one Kegel:

1. Sit in a comfortable chair, recliner, or sofa

2. Allow your mind to focus on your pelvic floor muscles.

3. Begin squeezing your bottom with your muscles. One of my patients, a photographer, thought of an analogy that

many of my patients find helpful. Think of your rectum like the shutter of a camera. Simply close the shutter with your mind.

4. Next imagine that your closed rectum is an elevator (another analogy). Quickly raise the elevator up towards your stomach.

5. Hold for a quick count of five (think "one, two, three, four, five," and NOT "one-Mississippi..."). Now bring it back down.

6. Allow your bottom to relax completely.

7. Repeat **at most** 10 times in quick succession. It should take you about 45-60 seconds, which means one second to raise the elevator, five quick-holding counts, and one second to lower it.

• The additional cough-Kegel

This week we add another Kegel at the end of each set of Kegels as described above. Here's how you do it:

1. Perform the Kegel while holding in your belly.

2. During the quick-holding step, produce an artificial cough. The reason for this is to get your body used to transient increases in intra-abdominal pressure, as coughing or sneezing does. These are times when you're more likely to leak, so we are intentionally simulating it to help you overcome this problem.

3. Note that this means you will be doing 8 extra cough-Kegels, because they are done after each set throughout the

day. Your total number of Kegels is up to 88 (80 holding Kegels and 8 cough-Kegels after each of 8 sets).

• Breathing and Other Exercises

This week you will continue two sets of the following exercises, once in the morning and once in the evening. Each set should now be 12 repetitions. For best results we also add an additional exercise involving a stretch band such as the Thera-Band®.

1. First begin with a set of deep breathing exercises:

–Breathe in through your nose and out through your mouth.

–Your exhale should be at least twice as long as your inhale; thus, if you breathe in for 3 seconds, breathe out for 6 seconds.

–Repeat the above 12 times total to complete the set.

Make sure you do not become lightheaded when doing these exercises; if you do, you are doing too many.

2. Next, move on to the set of leg rolls:

–Lie down on your back with your legs straight and spread apart by about 12 inches.

–Inhale slowly and roll both legs inward. At the same time gently squeeze your bottom and hold for a quick count of 3.

–Now exhale, roll both legs outward, and relax your bottom.

–Repeat the above 12 times total to complete the set.

3. The third exercise is the ball squeeze:

A few notes: It's most comfortable to do this exercise on a bed. You will need a soft, rubber ball. I highly recommend the cheap (usually under $2) 9-inch diameter balls at Walmart. Other balls, such as a football or basketball, are too sturdy.

–Lie down on your back with your knees bent and pointed upwards and feet flat on the bed.

–Place the ball between your knees.

–Inhale slowly while squeezing the ball and simultaneously squeezing your bottom (remember the elevator traveling towards your belly) for a quick count of 3.

–Release and repeat for a total of 12 times to complete the set.

4. The final exercise is basically the opposite of the ball squeeze and instead of adducting your legs you will be *abducting* them (moving them farther apart).

–Lie down on your back with your knees bent and pointed upwards and feet flat on the bed. Your legs can be close together at the starting position.

–Place the stretch band around both thighs, about 3 inches above your knees.

–Slowly move your knees apart about 8-10 inches, against the increasing tension in the band.

–Repeat this 12 times.

Expected Progress

Be sure you're keeping up with your bladder log so you can measure progress along the way. By the end of week three you should notice a few improvements:

–You should have minimal leakage while sleeping, as evidenced by a relatively dry pad when you wake up.

–If you do wake up at night to go to the restroom, you should notice that you can reach the toilet without leaking. Once you are there, the duration of your stream should be longer, meaning you have successfully voided.

–During the day you should also require fewer pads. For example, if a patient of mine uses 10 pads on Monday, by the following Sunday he may be using 7 pads. Ideally this decrease will be 30-50 percent. Don't forget, these are also smaller pads, so it's a double improvement.

Don't worry if you do not notice all of these changes immediately. People respond differently and some recover faster than others. The key is to be honest and consistent with sticking to the regiment—nutrition, exercises, and bladder log. If you have no appreciable improvements by this time, repeat week 3 until you notice an improvement before moving on to week 4.

• Take Home Points

I want to end this chapter in the same way that it began: with important points that deserve repetition because they are crucial to your recovery. Let us begin:

–Do not do Kegel exercises constantly; in fact, do not do more than 8 sets of 10 repetitions each day. Remember that the pelvic floor muscles are small, like the muscles of the hand or face, and thus, they fatigue quickly. When they are fatigued they cannot contract tightly, and when they cannot contract you leak more. **The more exercise you do past a certain point, the more you will leak!** This sounds opposite to what society teaches us: "No pain no gain."

−When you are sitting or walking make sure that you relax your rectum and perineal areas. My patients who worry about leaking often sit with them clenched, and thus, fatigue their pelvic floor muscles, leading to more leaking. The worry about leaking becomes a self-fulfilling prophecy!

−Do not try to stop the leakage right away; however, feel free to maintain a small amount of tension in your pelvic floor muscles. No matter what you do there will be at least some dribbling. It will stop. Give it time. It is a muscle. It takes at least 6-8 weeks to notice any changes after exercising other muscles, such as your abdominals or biceps, so remember that the same applies to your pelvic floor muscles. These muscles and the bladder will not strengthen and coordinate in a week!

That concludes the third week on your journey back to normalcy. You're a third of the way there! Celebrate your accomplishments thus far and stick with it.

Chapter Ten

Week Four—Heating Up

Introduction

You're almost half-way to the end of the program. Take a moment to pat yourself on the back. Conventional wisdom is that it takes three weeks for lifestyle changes to become habits. Though this is likely pretty variable depending upon the habit and personality, nonetheless, you should celebrate having made it this far.

I will continue repeating the most important points in each chapter to make sure they are truly driven home. Exercises require proper form, and diet should be closely followed to see the best results. These should be performed each day of the week for best results.

Must-Follow Advice

Exercise and muscles

- **At most** do eight (8) sets of Kegels each day.

    –DO NOT DO MORE. Doing more will fatigue your pelvic floor muscles, which then will not be able to contract, leading to you leaking more.

- Remember to **pull in your belly**.

The reason we pull in the abdomen (belly) is that the intra-abdominal pressure decreases. Also, if an ultrasound of the bladder is done when we pull in the belly, we are able to observe the bladder neck becoming slender, and therefore, the pelvic floor muscles—though weak—are able to tighten around the neck.

–Before standing up. Once you are up, let your belly relax gently, but do not let go completely so you do not leak too much. You may feel a dribble, which is perfectly normal at this stage. If you forget to pull in your belly before standing up, sit back down and immediately stand up again, this time with the correct form.

–Before sitting down. Once you are seated, relax gently.

–Before bending down. For example, to wipe your feet after a shower, pick something up from the floor, or put your shoes on.

• When sitting make sure your **bottom is relaxed**.

–If you sit with your bottom squeezed tightly, you will eventually feel pain in your rectal and genital areas. This will lead to increased leakage, again due to muscle fatigue.

–This is one reason deep breathing is such an important exercise. Breathe in through your lips, then as you breathe out, relax your bottom.

• **Breathe** on your way to the restroom.

–On your way to the restroom, blow small puffs of air through your mouth. Feel the air emerge over your lips. This relaxes your body and takes away your focus from leakage. It also maintains your pelvic floor muscles at an optimum tension; not too relaxed to cause leakage and not too contracted to cause fatigue.

Pad-Free Time

This week we continue the pad-free time, though modify it slightly to retrain your body so you understand how much tension in your pelvic floor is necessary to avoid leaking. You will need a wide mouthed jar, such as an empty peanut butter jar, or a small bucket before you begin this exercise.

After you perform your first set of morning exercises, remove your pad or other form of leakage protection. Then, while you are sitting down as per your normal routine—for example working on your computer or watching TV—do the following:

–Place a plastic bag, such as a garbage bag, on your seat and cover it with a hand towel or small square disposable mattress pad if you would prefer.

–Sit down wearing only your underwear. These will gradually become soaked, often within 30 minutes, but do not be alarmed. The reason this happens is that you have become used to the protection of the pad, and your mind does not notice or care as much about a damp pad but certainly feels the effect of wet underwear.

–An analogy would be getting in the habit of lifting a full bucket of water each day until your body learns to expect the weight of the full bucket. Then one day the bucket is only half-full but you lift it with the usual amount of force, surprising you when the water spills.

–Now for the modification. **Before you stand up** you will do two things: (1) place the jar under your penis so that if you leak it is caught in the container, and (2) do a Kegel while pulling in your belly. Now when you stand up you will leak immediately if you are either holding your belly and pelvic floor too tight or not tight enough. This position allows you to play around with the tension in your abdomen and pelvic floor to minimize the leak.

–Think of your sphincter as a tap with a bad washer. If you try to shut the tap too strongly there will be a gush of water. If you do not tighten it enough there will be a continuous dribble. But if you rotate the handle slowly you can stop the leak to the occasional few drops.

–The first time you do this, take two steps before you release the tension. The next day take three steps, and so forth until you reach week five. So say you take 2 steps on Monday and 3 steps on Tuesday, by that Sunday you should take 8 steps before letting go. Eventually, you should be able to make it all the way to the restroom without leaking.

–The purpose of this exercise is to get your mind and body used to returning to a pad-free lifestyle. Consistency is an important part of success, but dependency needs to be avoided.

Pad Protocol

–Use "Ultrathin" pads (heavy, medium or thin) so they will fit comfortably in your underwear.

–To wear, remove the sticky tape from under the pad and place inside of your Jockey underwear. Make sure that the underwear is not too tight when you put it on because the resulting discomfort may cause you to leak more.

–You will likely be changing your protective pads and Depends multiple times each day. Change them when they are soaked (generally 80% or more saturated) for consistency sake, and remember to keep track of how many you're using in the bladder log.

−Note: if your pad is too narrow and doesn't cover the base of your underwear, feel free to double up on them. You may go through them faster, but the eventual goal is to get you to be pad-free so you'll be saving in the long run—not to mention improving your quality of life—by doubling down and sticking to the regimen.

• Home Pad Use

This week, continue trying to reduce the size, absorbency (e.g. 2 or 3 dot), and number of pads you need to wear. If you feel comfortable, try any of these changes in the morning before switching back to larger or more absorbent pads in the afternoon and evening.

• Outside Pad Use

−Outside of the house try transitioning to a reduced absorbency pad (3 or 4 dots) such as the TENA Twist. Again, this may be frustrating initially, but we are trying to avoid making your body dependent on leakage protection.

−You can take extra pads with you in your bag or pocket.

−Feel free to check the pad as often as needed by taking restroom breaks, as frequently as each hour if you need to.

Exercise Protocol

• Important Points:

−Do not do more than eight (8) sets of Kegels each day. A set involves 10 repetitions.

–Within reason and until you are dry avoid BLT: bending, lifting, or twisting. Repetitive BLT movements while you are trying to recover your continence post-surgery may negatively influence the coordination and contractility of the pelvic floor muscles and sphincter. In addition, intra-abdominal pressure increases when we bend, lift, or twist and the pelvic floor muscles are not yet strong enough to counteract this.

–Try not to lift anything more than 8-10 pounds in weight. That means laying off heavy housework, including but not limited to scrubbing, mopping with a cloth mop, vacuuming with a cleaner that is not self-propelled, cleaning the garage, polishing the car, remodeling the bathroom, and picking weeds. Note that this is **not a permanent** prescription, which your spouse may be happy to know!

–Do not perform abdominal, endurance, and free weight exercises while recovering this week. The only acceptable form of exercise is walking at a slow pace.

–You can do some BLT such as putting your shoes and pants on, feeding your pet, and taking clothes out of the washer/dryer.

• Kegels

Note that the Kegel protocol changes slightly each week so it will be important for you to follow the specific steps below while keeping in mind the general form of the exercises as described in an earlier chapter.

–The first step before performing your Kegels is to update your bladder log. Remember that this should become a daily habit so that you keep track of your progress over time.

–Next get into position and practice one Kegel:

1. Sit in a comfortable chair, recliner, or sofa

2. Allow your mind to focus on your pelvic floor muscles.

3. Begin squeezing your bottom with your muscles. One of my patients, a photographer, thought of an analogy that many of my patients find helpful. Think of your rectum like the shutter of a camera. Simply close the shutter with your mind.

4. Next imagine that your closed rectum is an elevator (another analogy). Quickly raise the elevator up towards your stomach.

5. Hold for a quick count of five (think "one, two, three, four, five," and NOT "one-Mississippi…"). Now bring it back down.

6. Allow your bottom to relax completely.

7. Repeat **at most** 10 times in quick succession. It should take you about 45-60 seconds, which means one second to raise the elevator, five quick-holding counts, and one second to lower it.

• The additional cough-Kegel

We continue the cough-Kegel at the end of each set of Kegels as described above. Here's a reminder on how to do it:

1. Perform the Kegel while holding in your belly.

2. During the quick-holding step, produce an artificial cough. The reason for this is to get your body used to transient

increases in intra-abdominal pressure, as coughing or sneezing does. These are times when you're more likely to leak, so we are intentionally simulating it to help you overcome this problem.

3. Note that this means you will be doing 8 extra cough-Kegels, because they are done after each set throughout the day. Your total number of Kegels is up to 88 (80 holding Kegels and 8 cough-Kegels after each of 8 sets).

• Breathing and Other Exercises

This week you will continue two sets of the following exercises, once in the morning and once in the evening. Each set should still be 12 repetitions. Since you're becoming stronger this week there is another exercise: the reverse abdominals.

1. First begin with a set of deep breathing exercises:

– Breathe in through your nose and out through your mouth.

–Your exhale should be at least twice as long as your inhale; thus, if you breathe in for 3 seconds, breathe out for 6 seconds.

–Repeat the above 12 times total to complete the set.

–Make sure you do not become lightheaded when doing these exercises; if you do, you are doing too many.

2. Next move on to the set of leg rolls:

–Lie down on your back with your legs straight and spread apart by about 12 inches.

–Inhale slowly and roll both legs inward. At the same time gently squeeze your bottom and hold for a quick count of 3.

–Now exhale, roll both legs outward, and relax your bottom.

–Repeat the above 12 times total to complete the set.

3. The third exercise is the ball squeeze:

A few notes: It's most comfortable to do this exercise on a bed. You will need a soft, rubber ball. I highly recommend the cheap (usually under $2) 9-inch diameter balls at Walmart. Other balls, such as a football or basketball, are too sturdy.

–Lie down on your back with your knees bent and pointed upwards and feet flat on the bed.

–Place the ball between your knees.

–Inhale slowly while squeezing the ball and simultaneously squeezing your bottom (remember the elevator traveling towards your belly) for a quick count of 3.

–Release and repeat for a total of 12 times to complete the set.

4. The fourth exercise is basically the opposite of the ball squeeze and instead of adducting your legs you will be abducting them (moving them farther apart).

–Lie down on your back with your knees bent and pointed upwards and feet flat on the bed. Your legs can be close together at the starting position.

–Place the stretch band around both thighs, about 3 inches above your knees.

–Slowly move your knees apart about 8-10 inches, against the increasing tension in the band. Hold for a quick count of 3.

−Repeat this 12 times.

5. The fifth exercise is the reverse abdominal.

−Lie on your back and bend both of your knees. Place your hands around one of your knees.

−Now lift that leg up so that your thigh is 90 degrees to the surface you're lying on and your knee is perpendicular to your thigh. Then bring the knee to your chest, while your hands gently push back to provide resistance. Hold for a quick count of 3.

−Repeat with the other leg. Doing both legs counts as one overall repetition, and you should do two sets of five repetitions each day.

6. **The restroom exercise**. If you want to recover even sooner, here's a secret exercise that you can incorporate into your restroom breaks.

−After you're finished on the toilet, sit with your back straight, count to 30 seconds, then lean forward and push like you are releasing gas. Repeat for a total of two times.

−The point of this is to "double-void" and empty the bladder out completely, so there is no residual urine left. This gets your body in the habit of complete emptying, which is important to prevent leakage and accidents after standing up.

Expected Progress

By the end of week 4 you should be able to get up in the night when you need to use the restroom without leaking. It should be natural like it was prior to surgery. Another sign of progress that you should notice is that you will be barely wet at night (maybe 10%). Assuming that you have no other sleeping difficulties, you should notice that you are sleeping for longer periods of time.

• Take Home Points

I want to end this chapter in the same way that it began: with important points that deserve repetition because they are crucial to your recovery. Let us begin:

–Do not do Kegel exercises constantly; in fact, do not do more than 8 sets of 10 repetitions each day. Remember that the pelvic floor muscles are small, like the muscles of the hand or face, and thus, they fatigue quickly. When they are fatigued they cannot contract tightly, and when they cannot contract, you leak more. **The more exercise you do past a certain point, the more you will leak!** This sounds opposite to what society teaches us: "No pain no gain."

–When you are sitting or walking make sure that you relax your rectum and perineal areas. My patients who worry about leaking often sit with them clenched, and thus, fatigue their pelvic floor muscles, leading to more leaking. The worry about leaking becomes a self-fulfilling prophecy!

–Do not try to stop the leakage right away; however, feel free to maintain a small amount of tension in your pelvic floor muscles. No matter what you do there will be at least some dribbling. It will stop. Give it time. It is a muscle. It takes at least 6-8 weeks to notice any changes after exercising other muscles, such as your abdominals or biceps, so remember that the same applies to your pelvic floor muscles. These muscles and the bladder will not strengthen and coordinate in a week!

That concludes the fourth week on your journey back to normalcy. You're half-way there! Celebrate your accomplishments thus far and stay the course!

Chapter Eleven

Week Five—Over the Hump

Introduction

You've reached the midway point! By now you should certainly be seeing at least small improvements, such as less frequent accidents or longer stream durations. Just *keep on keeping on*, because the best has yet to come!

I will continue repeating the most important points in each chapter to make sure they are truly driven home. Exercises require proper form, and diet should be closely followed to see the best results. These should be performed each day of the week for best results.

Must-Follow Advice

Exercise and Muscles

- **At most** do eight (8) sets of Kegels each day.

  –DO NOT DO MORE. Doing more will fatigue your pelvic floor muscles, which then will not be able to contract, leading to you leaking more.

- Remember to pull in your belly.

The reason we pull in the abdomen (belly) is that the intra-abdominal pressure decreases. Also, if an ultrasound of the bladder is done when we pull in the belly, we are able to observe the bladder neck becoming slender, and therefore, the pelvic floor muscles—though weak—are able to tighten around the neck.

−Before standing up. Once you are up, let your belly relax gently, but do not let go completely so you do not leak too much. You may feel a dribble, which is perfectly normal at this stage. If you forget to pull in your belly before standing up, sit back down and immediately stand up again, this time with the correct form.

−Before sitting down. Once you are seated, relax gently.

−Before bending down. For example, to wipe your feet after a shower, pick something up from the floor, or put your shoes on.

• When sitting make sure your **bottom is relaxed**.

−If you sit with your bottom squeezed tightly, you will eventually feel pain in your rectal and genital areas. This will lead to increased leakage, again due to muscle fatigue.

−This is one reason deep breathing is such an important exercise. Breathe in through your lips, then as you breathe out, relax your bottom.

• When standing make sure your **bottom is relaxed**.

−Whenever you are standing for extended periods of time—for example, waiting in line at the grocery store—make sure that your rectal and genital area is relaxed. People tend to constantly be clenching because they are afraid to leak.

−The best way I've found for having my patients relax is to have them pretend to pass gas for a quick count of three, which will then help them relax their bottom and overall decrease muscle fatigue.

● **Breathe** on your way to the restroom.

–On your way to the restroom, blow small puffs of air through your mouth. Feel the air emerge over your lips. This relaxes your body and takes away your focus from leakage. It also maintains your pelvic floor muscles at an optimum tension— not too relaxed to cause leakage and not too contracted to cause fatigue.

Pad-Free Time

This week we continue the pad-free time with the slight modification to retrain your body so you understand how much tension in your pelvic floor is necessary to avoid leaking. You will need a wide mouthed jar, such as an empty peanut butter jar, or a small bucket before you begin this exercise.

After you perform your first set of morning exercises, remove your pad or other form of leakage protection. Then, while you are sitting down as per your normal routine—for example working on your computer or watching TV—do the following:

–Place a plastic bag, such as a garbage bag, on your seat and cover it with a hand towel or small square disposable mattress pad if you would prefer.

–Sit down wearing only your underwear. These will gradually become soaked, often within 30 minutes, but do not be alarmed. The reason this happens is that you have become used to the protection of the pad, and your mind does not notice or care as much about a damp pad but certainly feels the effect of wet underwear.

a. An analogy would be getting in the habit of lifting a full bucket of water each day until your body learns to expect

121

the weight of the full bucket. Then one day the bucket is only half-full but you lift it with the usual amount of force, surprising you when the water spills.

–Before you stand up you will do two things: (1) place the jar under your penis so that if you leak it is caught in the container, and (2) do a Kegel while pulling in your belly. Now when you stand up you will leak immediately if you are either holding your belly and pelvic floor too tight or not tight enough. This position allows you to play around with the tension in your abdomen and pelvic floor to minimize the leak.

–The first time you do this, take two steps before you release the tension. The next day take three steps, and so forth until you reach week five. So say you take 2 steps on Monday and 3 steps on Tuesday, by that Sunday you should take 8 steps before letting go. Eventually, you should be able to make it all the way to the restroom without leaking.

–The purpose of this exercise is to get your mind and body used to returning to a pad-free lifestyle. Consistency is an important part success, but dependency needs to be avoided.

Pad Protocol

–Use "Ultrathin" pads (heavy, medium or thin) so they will fit comfortably in your underwear.

–To wear, remove the sticky tape from under the pad and place inside of your Jockey underwear. Make sure that the underwear is not too tight when you put it on because the resulting discomfort may cause you to leak more.

–You will likely be changing your protective pads and Depends multiple times each day. Change them when they are soaked (generally 80% or more saturated) for consistency sake, and remember to keep track of how many you're using in the bladder log.

–Note: If your pad is too narrow and doesn't cover the base of your underwear, feel free to double up on them. You may go through them faster, but the eventual goal is to get you to be pad-free so you'll be saving in the long run—not to mention improving your quality of life—by doubling down and sticking to the regimen.

• Home Pad Use

–This week, continue trying to reduce the size, absorbency (e.g. 2 or 3 dot), and number of pads you need to wear. Ideally, you can wear a lighter pad consistently throughout the day.

–If you are waking up in the morning without much leakage, you can stop using pads while you sleep. I know it's comforting to have leak protection, but remember what we've said about becoming dependent.

• Outside Pad Use

–Outside of the house make the full transition to a reduced absorbency pad (3 or 4 dots), such as the TENA Twist.

–Hopefully, you will be taking a fewer number of extra pads with you in your bag or pocket and your need to check them has reduced.

Exercise Protocol

• Important Points:

–Do not do more than eight (8) sets of Kegels each day. A set involves 10 repetitions.

–Within reason and until you are dry avoid BLT: bending, lifting, or twisting. Repetitive BLT movements while you are trying to recover your continence post-surgery may negatively influence the coordination and contractility of the pelvic floor muscles and sphincter. In addition, intra-abdominal pressure increases when we bend, lift, or twist and the pelvic floor muscles are not yet strong enough to counteract this.

–Try not to lift anything more than 8-10 pounds in weight. That means laying off heavy housework, including but not limited to scrubbing, mopping with a cloth mop, vacuuming with a cleaner that is not self-propelled, cleaning the garage, polishing the car, remodeling the bathroom, and picking weeds. Note that this is **not a permanent** prescription, which your spouse may be happy to know!

–Do not perform abdominal, endurance, and free weight exercises while recovering this week. The only acceptable form of exercise is walking at a slow pace.

–You can do some BLT such as putting your shoes and pants on, feeding your pet, and taking clothes out of the washer/dryer.

• Kegels

Note that the Kegel protocol changes slightly each week so it will be important for you to follow the specific steps below while keeping in mind the general form of the exercises as described in an earlier chapter.

–The first step before performing your Kegels is to update your bladder log. Remember that this should become a daily habit so that you keep track of your progress over time.

−Next get into position and practice one Kegel:

1. Sit in a comfortable chair, recliner, or sofa

2. Allow your mind to focus on your pelvic floor muscles.

3. Begin squeezing your bottom with your muscles. One of my patients, a photographer, thought of an analogy that many of my patients find helpful. Think of your rectum like the shutter of a camera. Simply close the shutter with your mind.

4. Next imagine that your closed rectum is an elevator (another analogy courtesy of a patient). Quickly raise the elevator up towards your stomach.

5. **Important addition**. Note that the Kegel protocol has changed this week. While you are holding in the next step, you will simultaneously tighten your penis and scrotum by imagining that you are trying to prevent yourself from urinating. Thus, your entire pelvic region will be tightened for the count.

6. Hold for a quick count of five (think "one, two, three, four, five," and NOT "one-Mississippi..."). Now bring it back down.

7. Allow your bottom to relax completely.

8. Repeat **at most** 10 times in quick succession. It should take you about 45-60 seconds, which means one second to raise the elevator, five quick-holding counts, and one second to lower it.

•The additional cough-Kegel

We continue the cough-Kegel at the end of each set of Kegels as described above. Here's a reminder on how to do it:

–Perform the Kegel while holding in your belly.

–During the quick-holding step, produce an artificial cough. The reason for this is to get your body used to transient increases in intra-abdominal pressure, as coughing or sneezing does. These are times when you're more likely to leak, so we are intentionally simulating it to help you overcome this problem.

–Note that this means you will be doing 8 extra cough-Kegels because they are done after each set throughout the day. Your total number of Kegels is up to 88 (80 holding Kegels and 8 cough-Kegels after each of 8 sets).

• Breathing and Other Exercises

This week you will continue two sets of the following exercises, once in the morning and once in the evening. Each set should still be 12 repetitions. Since you're becoming stronger, this week there is another exercise: the leg lift.

1. First begin with a set of deep breathing exercises:

–Breathe in through your nose and out through your mouth.

–Your exhale should be at least twice as long as your inhale; thus, if you breathe in for 3 seconds, breathe out for 6 seconds.

–Repeat the above 12 times total to complete the set.

Make sure you do not become lightheaded when doing these exercises; if you do, you are doing too many.

2. Next, move on to the set of leg rolls:

   –Lie down on your back with your legs straight and spread apart by about 12 inches.

   –Inhale slowly and roll both legs inward. At the same time, gently squeeze your bottom and hold for a quick count of 5 (**Note the increased holding length here).**

   –Now exhale, roll both legs outward, and relax your bottom.

   –Repeat the above 12 times total to complete the set.

3. The third exercise is the ball squeeze.

It's most comfortable to do this exercise on a bed. You will need a soft, rubber ball. I highly recommend the cheap (usually under $2) 9-inch diameter balls at Walmart. Other balls, such as a football or basketball, are too sturdy.

   –Lie down on your back with your knees bent and pointed upwards and feet flat on the bed.

   –Place the ball between your knees.

   –Inhale slowly while squeezing the ball and simultaneously squeezing your bottom (remember the elevator traveling towards your belly) for a quick count of five.

   –Release and repeat for a total of 12 times to complete the set.

4. The fourth exercise is basically the opposite of the ball squeeze and instead of adducting your legs you will be abducting them (moving them farther apart).

–Lie down on your back with your knees bent and pointed upwards and feet flat on the bed. Your legs can be close together at the starting position.

–Place the stretch band around both thighs, about 3 inches above your knees.

–Slowly move your knees apart about 8-10 inches, against the increasing tension in the band. Hold for a quick count of 5.

–Repeat this 12 times.

5. The fifth exercise is the reverse abdominal.

–Lie on your back and bend both of your knees. Place your hands around one of your knees.

–Now lift that leg up so that your thigh is 90 degrees to the surface you're lying on and your knee is perpendicular to your thigh. Then bring the knee to your chest, while your hands gently push back to provide resistance. Hold for a quick count of five.

–Complete 5 repetitions to finish the set before switching over to the other leg and doing the same. Remember to do two sets each day: morning and evening.

6. The sixth exercise is the leg lift. This also works out your abdominals. This exercise and the one above are preferable to crunches because crunches increase the abdominal pressure more significantly, potentially leading to increased leaking.

–Lie on your back with one leg bent and the other straightened on the surface.

–Raise the straight leg up to about 70 degrees. Hold it for a quick count of five then bring it down.

–Complete 5 repetitions to finish the set before switching over to the other leg and doing the same. Remember to do two sets each day: morning and evening.

7. **The restroom exercise.** If you want to recover even sooner, here's a secret exercise that you can incorporate into your restroom breaks.

–After you're finished on the toilet, sit with your back straight, count to 30 seconds, then lean forward and push like you are releasing gas. Repeat for a total of two times.

–The point of this is to "double-void" and empty the bladder out completely, so there is no residual urine left. This gets your body in the habit of complete emptying, which is important to prevent leakage and accidents after standing up.

Expected Progress

By the end of week five you should notice a few significant improvements, such as the ability to:

–Sit without a pad for more than two hours.

–Sleep without a pad at night and still be dry.

–Make it to the bathroom in the morning without leaking, and every hour or so thereafter. Your stream will still be short.

–Wear two-dot pads at home which get about 50% wet, and no longer completely soaked.

• Take Home Points

I want to end this chapter in the same way that it began: with important points that deserve repetition because they are crucial to your recovery. Let us begin:

–Do not do Kegel exercises constantly; in fact, do not do more than 8 sets of 10 repetitions each day. Remember that the pelvic floor muscles are small, like the muscles of the hand or face, and thus, they fatigue quickly. When they are fatigued they cannot contract tightly, and when they cannot contract you leak more. **The more exercise you do past a certain point, the more you will leak!** This sounds opposite to what society teaches us: "No pain no gain."

–When you are sitting or walking make sure that you relax your rectum and perineal areas. My patients who worry about leaking often sit with them clenched, and thus, fatigue their pelvic floor muscles, leading to more leaking. The worry about leaking becomes a self-fulfilling prophecy!

–Do not try to stop the leakage right away; however, feel free to maintain a small amount of tension in your pelvic floor muscles. No matter what you do there will be at least some dribbling. It will stop. Give it time. It is a muscle. It takes at least 6-8 weeks to notice any changes after exercising other muscles, such as your abdominals or biceps, so remember that the same applies to your pelvic floor muscles. These muscles and the bladder will not strengthen and coordinate in a week!

That concludes the fifth week on your journey back to normalcy. Celebrate your accomplishments thus far and stay the course!

Chapter Twelve

Week Six—Dry at Night

Introduction

Congratulations on making it over the first hump. You're going to continue working hard with the base routine you've established by now, and this week we're going to pick up the pace by adding a few major modifications.

As always, *I will continue repeating the most important points in each chapter to make sure they are truly driven home.* Exercises require proper form, and diet should be closely followed to see the best results. These should be performed each day of the week for best results.

Must-Follow Advice

Exercise and Muscles

- **At most** do eight (8) sets of Kegels each day.

   –DO NOT DO MORE. Doing more will fatigue your pelvic floor muscles, which then will not be able to contract leading to you leaking more.

- Remember to **pull in your belly**.

The reason we pull in the abdomen (belly) is that the intra-abdominal pressure decreases. Also, if an ultrasound of the bladder is done when we pull in the belly, we are able to observe the bladder neck becoming slender, and therefore, the pelvic floor muscles—though weak—are able to tighten around the neck.

–Before standing up. Once you are up, let your belly relax gently, but do not let go completely so you do not leak too much. You may feel a dribble, which is perfectly normal at this stage. If you forget to pull in your belly before standing up, sit back down and immediately stand up again, this time with the correct form.

–Before sitting down. Once you are seated, relax gently.

–Before bending down. For example, to wipe your feet after a shower, pick something up from the floor, or put your shoes on.

• When sitting make sure your **bottom is relaxed**.

–If you sit with your bottom squeezed tightly, you will eventually feel pain in your rectal and genital areas. This will lead to increased leakage, again due to muscle fatigue.

–This is one reason deep breathing is such an important exercise. Breathe in through your lips, then as you breathe out, relax your bottom.

• When standing make sure your **bottom is relaxed**.

–Whenever you are standing for extended periods of time—for example, waiting in line at the grocery store—make sure that your rectal and genital area is relaxed. People tend to constantly be clenching because they are afraid to leak.

–The best way I've found for having my patients relax is to have them pretend to pass gas for a quick count of three, which will then help them relax their bottom and overall decrease muscle fatigue.

- **Breathe** on your way to the restroom.

    −On your way to the restroom, blow small puffs of air through your mouth. Feel the air emerge over your lips. This relaxes your body and takes away your focus from leakage. It also maintains your pelvic floor muscles at an optimum tension; not too relaxed to cause leakage and not too contracted to cause fatigue.

- Pad-Free Time

This week we continue the pad-free time with the slight modification to retrain your body so you understand how much tension in your pelvic floor is necessary to avoid leaking. You will need a wide mouthed jar, such as an empty peanut butter jar, or a small bucket before you begin this exercise.

    −By now you will notice that you can control the stream until you reach the restroom. Barely anything should leak out of the jar, and if that is the case, you can stop using a jar.

After you perform your first set of morning exercises, remove your pad or other form of leakage protection. Then, while you are sitting down as per your normal routine—for example, working on your computer or watching TV—do the following:

    −Place a plastic bag, such as a garbage bag, on your seat and cover it with a hand towel or small square disposable mattress pad if you would prefer.

    −Sit down wearing only your underwear. These will gradually become soaked, often within 30 minutes, but do not be alarmed. The reason this happens is that you have become used to the protection of the pad, and your mind does not notice or care as much about a damp pad but certainly feels the effect of wet underwear.

> a. An analogy would be getting in the habit of lifting a full bucket of water each day until your body learns to expect the weight of the full bucket. Then one day the bucket is only half-full but you lift it with the usual amount of force, surprising you when the water spills.

—Before you stand up you will do two things: (1) place the jar under your penis so that if you leak it is caught in the container, and (2) do a Kegel while pulling in your belly. Now when you stand up, you will leak immediately if you are either holding your belly and pelvic floor too tight or not tight enough. This position allows you to play around with the tension in your abdomen and pelvic floor to minimize the leak.

—The first time you do this, take two steps before you release the tension. The next day take three steps, and so forth until you reach week five. So say you take 2 steps on Monday and 3 steps on Tuesday, by that Sunday you should take 8 steps before letting go. Eventually, you should be able to make it all the way to the restroom without leaking.

—The purpose of this exercise is to get your mind and body used to returning to a pad-free lifestyle. Consistency is an important part success, but dependency needs to be avoided.

Pad Protocol

—Use "Ultrathin" pads (heavy, medium or thin) so they will fit comfortably in your underwear.

–Make sure that the pads are "Ultrathin" so they will fit comfortably in your underwear.

–To wear, remove the sticky tape from under the pad and place inside of your Jockey underwear. Make sure that the underwear is not too tight when you put it on because the resulting discomfort may cause you to leak more.

–You will likely be changing your protective pads and Depends multiple times each day. Change them when they are soaked (generally 80% or more saturated) for consistency sake, and remember to keep track of how many you're using in the bladder log.

–Note: if your pad is too narrow and doesn't cover the base of your underwear, feel free to double up on them. You may go through them faster, but the eventual goal is to get you to be pad-free so you'll be saving in the long run—not to mention improving your quality of life—by doubling down and sticking to the regimen.

• Home Pad Use

–We have reached an inflection point this week. At this point you should not be using pads as you sleep because you are not leaking overnight.

–In the morning you can begin using pantyliners. Unfortunately, my patients have not found better options for men, so pantyliners have to do. There are also many different brands available for these.

–During the rest of the day at home you can be using ultrathin light absorbency pads (1 dot).

• Outside Pad Use

This week I want to draw a distinction between going out for short trips to the store, post office, neighbor's house, etc. and longer trips that require you to be out for longer than an hour. Your leak protection strategy will differ depending on which type of trip you are taking.

–On quick trips you can start using ultrathin light absorbency pads (1 dot). These trips should be under 30 minutes. For example, to pick up milk from the local grocer or mail a letter at the post office.

–On longer trips, such as shopping at the mall or socializing at a party, you should be using slightly heavier pads (2 dots). Fortunately, in America we are never too far away from the porcelain throne, and so you can almost always change your pad in a restroom if you leaked. Remember to take along extra pads, and make sure to change the one you are wearing if it gets more than half-soaked.

Exercise Protocol

• Important Points:

–Do not do more than eight (8) sets of Kegels each day. A set involves 10 repetitions.

–Within reason and until you are dry avoid BLT: bending, lifting, or twisting. Repetitive BLT movements while you are trying to recover your continence post-surgery may negatively influence the coordination and contractility of the pelvic floor muscles and sphincter. In addition, intra-abdominal pressure increases when we bend, lift, or twist and the pelvic floor muscles are not yet strong enough to counteract this.

−Try not to lift anything more than 8-10 pounds in weight. That means laying off heavy housework, including but not limited to scrubbing, mopping with a cloth mop, vacuuming with a cleaner that is not self-propelled, cleaning the garage, polishing the car, remodeling the bathroom, and picking weeds. Note that this is **not a permanent** prescription, which your spouse may be happy to know!

−Do not perform abdominal, endurance, and free weight exercises while recovering this week. The only acceptable form of exercise is walking at a slow pace.

−You can do some BLT such as putting your shoes and pants on, feeding your pet, and taking clothes out of the washer/dryer.

- Kegels

  −Note that the Kegel protocol changes slightly each week so it will be important for you to follow the specific steps below while keeping in mind the general form of the exercises as described in an earlier chapter.

  −The first step before performing your Kegels is to update your bladder log. Remember that this should become a daily habit so that you keep track of your progress over time.

  −This week is the most significant change to the Kegel protocol since we started. We make a distinction between the complete Kegel, which involves tightening both your bottom (shutter/elevator) and your frontal (stop urinating mid-stream) pelvic floor muscles. You will still complete 8 sets, but alternate between a set of complete and a set of frontal-only Kegels.

–Thus, if you begin your Kegels at 6 am, an example schedule would be as follows:

- 6 am - set of complete Kegels with cough Kegel
- 8 am - set of frontal Kegel with cough Kegel
- 10 am - set of complete Kegels with cough Kegel
- 12 pm - set of frontal Kegel with cough Kegel
- And so forth until 8 sets have been completed

–Let's begin:

1. Performing a complete Kegel:

–Sit in a comfortable chair, recliner, or sofa

–Allow your mind to focus on your pelvic floor muscles.

–Begin squeezing your bottom with your muscles. One of my patients, a photographer, thought of an analogy that many of my patients find helpful. Think of your rectum like the shutter of a camera. Simply close the shutter with your mind.

–Next imagine that your closed rectum is an elevator (another analogy). Quickly raise the elevator up towards your stomach.

–While you are holding in the next step, you will simultaneously tighten your penis and scrotum by imagining that you are trying to prevent yourself from urinating. Thus, your entire pelvic region will be tightened for the count.

–**Hold for a quick count of five** (think "one, two, three, four, five," and NOT "one-Mississippi..."). Now bring it back down.

–Allow your bottom to relax completely.

–Repeat **at most** 10 times in quick succession. It should take you about 45-60 seconds, which means one second to raise the elevator, five quick-holding counts, and one second to lower it.

2. Performing a frontal Kegel

–The frontal Kegel is faster because it only involves tightening the frontal pelvic floor muscles. You can do this by imagining that you are stopping urination mid-stream.

–You should do these quickly and be able to complete 10 repetitions within 20 seconds.

3. **The additional cough-Kegel.**

We continue the cough-Kegel at the end of each set of Kegels as described above. Here's a reminder on how to do it:

–Perform the Kegel while holding in your belly.

–During the quick-holding step, produce an artificial cough. The reason for this is to get your body used to transient increases in intra-abdominal pressure, as coughing or sneezing does. These are times when you're more likely to leak, so we are intentionally simulating it to help you overcome this problem.

–Note that this means you will be doing 8 extra cough-Kegels because they are done after each set throughout the day. Your total number of Kegels is up to 88 (80 holding Kegels and 8 cough-Kegels after each of 8 sets).

• Breathing and Other Exercises

–This week you will continue two sets of the following exercises, once in the morning and once in the evening. Each set should still be 15 repetitions. Since you're becoming stronger, this week there is another exercise: the feet lift.

1. First begin with a set of deep breathing exercises:

—Breathe in through your nose and out through your mouth.

—Your exhale should be at least twice as long as your inhale; thus, if you breathe in for 3 seconds, breathe out for 6 seconds.

—Repeat the above 15 times total to complete the set.

Make sure you do not become lightheaded when doing these exercises; if you do, you are doing too many.

2. Next move on to the set of leg rolls:

—Lie down on your back with your legs straight and spread apart by about 12 inches.

—Inhale slowly and roll both legs inward. At the same time gently squeeze your bottom and hold for a quick count of five.

—Now exhale, roll both legs outward, and relax your bottom.

—Repeat the above 15 times total to complete the set.

3. The third exercise is the ball squeeze:

A few notes: It's most comfortable to do this exercise on a bed.

You will need a soft, rubber ball. I highly recommend the cheap (usually under $2) 9-inch diameter balls at Walmart. Other balls, such as a football or basketball, are too sturdy.

–Lie down on your back with your knees bent and pointed upwards and feet flat on the bed.

–Place the ball between your knees.

–Inhale slowly while squeezing the ball and simultaneously squeezing your bottom (remember the elevator traveling towards your belly) for a quick count of five.

–Release and repeat for a total of 15 times to complete the set.

4. The fourth exercise is basically the opposite of the ball squeeze and instead of adducting your legs you will be abducting them (moving them farther apart).

–Lie down on your back with your knees bent and pointed upwards and feet flat on the bed. Your legs can be close together at the starting position.

–Place the stretch band around both thighs, about 3 inches above your knees.

–Slowly move your knees apart about 8-10 inches, against the increasing tension in the band. Hold for a quick count of five.

–Repeat this 15 times.

5. The fifth exercise is the reverse abdominal.

–Lie on your back and bend both of your knees. Place your hands around one of your knees.

–Now lift that leg up so that your thigh is 90 degrees to the surface you're lying on and your knee is perpendicular to your thigh. Then bring the knee to your chest, while your hands gently push back to provide resistance. Hold for a quick count of five.

–Complete five repetitions to finish the set before switching over to the other leg and doing the same. Remember to do two sets each day: morning and evening.

6. The sixth exercise is the leg lift. This also works out your abdominals. This exercise and the one above are preferable to crunches because crunches increase the abdominal pressure more significantly, potentially leading to increased leaking.

–Lie on your back with one leg bent and the other straightened on the surface.

–Raise the straight leg up to about 70 degrees. Hold it for a quick count of five then bring it down.

–Complete five repetitions to finish the set before switching over to the other leg and doing the same. Remember to do two sets each day: morning and evening.

7. The seventh exercise, also targeting the abdominals, is the feet lift.

–Similar to the exercises above, lie flat on your back with both legs bent and your feet flat on the surface.

–Lift **both** feet simultaneously so that your thighs are perpendicular to the surface and your lower legs are parallel to it.

–Hold for a quick count of five, and repeat five times total to complete the set.

8. The restroom exercise. If you want to recover even sooner, here's a secret exercise that you can incorporate into your restroom breaks.

–After you're finished on the toilet, sit with your back straight, count to 30 seconds, then lean forward and push like you are releasing gas. Repeat for a total of two times.

–The point of this is to "double-void" and empty the bladder out completely, so there is no residual urine left. This gets your body in the habit of complete emptying, which is important to prevent leakage and accidents after standing up.

Expected Progress

After week six you should notice the following:

–You are almost dry till mid-morning. In the evening after 5 or 6 pm you should also be dry, especially if you decrease your activity.

–The afternoon, e.g. 2-4 pm, will be your most leaky period, but we'll decrease that soon enough.

–You are using fewer one-dot pads at home, perhaps one every two hours. This equates to about a tablespoon of leakage. Much better!

• Take Home Points

I want to end this chapter in the same way that it began: with important points that deserve repetition because they are crucial to your recovery. Let us begin:

–Do not do Kegel exercises constantly; in fact, do not do more than 8 sets of 10 repetitions each day. Remember that the pelvic floor muscles are small, like the muscles of the hand or face, and thus, they fatigue quickly. When they are fatigued they cannot contract tightly, and when they cannot contract you leak more. **The more exercise you do past a certain point, the more you will leak!** This sounds opposite to what society teaches us: "No pain no gain."

–When you are sitting or walking make sure that you relax your rectum and perineal areas. My patients who worry about leaking often sit with them clenched, and thus, fatigue their pelvic floor muscles, leading to more leaking. The worry about leaking becomes a self-fulfilling prophecy!

–Do not try to stop the leakage right away; however, feel free to maintain a small amount of tension in your pelvic floor muscles. No matter what you do there will be at least some dribbling. It will stop. Give it time. It is a muscle. It takes at least 6-8 weeks to notice any changes after exercising other muscles, such as your abdominals or biceps, so remember that the same applies to your pelvic floor muscles. These muscles and the bladder will not strengthen and coordinate in a week!

–By this week you should be noticing some good progress in how much you're leaking and able to control accidents. If there are still significant issues, which there may be because everyone is different, here are a few important trouble-shooting tips:

−Drink lots of water to avoid getting dehydrated. Remember our discussion on that earlier in the book. Milk is fine to drink as well, though stay away from artificial sweeteners and acidic beverages.

−Avoid highly processed foods like TV dinners. Too much sugar, salt, or preservatives can aggravate the bladder and promote leakage.

−If you are leaking, perform the pushing out the wind exercise for a quick count of three every half-hour or so.

−Remember to relax your pelvic floor muscles while sitting or standing. The more constantly fatigued they are the more you will leak.

That concludes the sixth week on your journey back to normalcy. Celebrate your accomplishments thus far and be consistent so you don't have to be dependent.

Chapter Thirteen

Week Seven—Dry in the Morning

Introduction

You're two-thirds of the way there! By now you should be seeing some noticeable improvements in your continence.

As always, *I will continue repeating the most important points in each chapter to make sure they are truly driven home*. Exercises require proper form, and diet should be closely followed to see the best results. These should be performed each day of the week for best results.

Must-Follow Advice

Exercise and Muscles

- **At most** do eight (8) sets of Kegels each day.

  –DO NOT DO MORE. Doing more will fatigue your pelvic floor muscles, which then will not be able to contract, leading to you leaking more.

- Remember to **pull in your belly**.

The reason we pull in the abdomen (belly) is that the intra-abdominal pressure decreases. Also, if an ultrasound of the bladder is done when we pull in the belly, we are able to observe the bladder neck becoming slender, and therefore, the pelvic floor muscles—though weak—are able to tighten around the neck.

−Before standing up. Once you are up, let your belly relax gently, but do not let go completely so you do not leak too much. You may feel a dribble, which is perfectly normal at this stage. If you forget to pull in your belly before standing up, sit back down and immediately stand up again, this time with the correct form.

−Before sitting down. Once you are seated, relax gently.

−Before bending down. For example, to wipe your feet after a shower, pick something up from the floor, or put your shoes on.

• When sitting make sure your **bottom is relaxed**.

−If you sit with your bottom squeezed tightly, you will eventually feel pain in your rectal and genital areas. This will lead to increased leakage, again due to muscle fatigue.

−This is one reason deep breathing is such an important exercise. Breathe in through your lips, then as you breathe out, relax your bottom.

• When standing make sure your **bottom is relaxed**.

−Whenever you are standing for extended periods of time—for example, waiting in line at the grocery store—make sure that your rectal and genital area is relaxed. People tend to constantly be clenching because they are afraid to leak.

−The best way I've found for having my patients relax is to have them pretend to pass gas for a quick count of three, which will then help them relax their bottom and overall decrease muscle fatigue.

- **Breathe** on your way to the restroom.

  −On your way to the restroom, blow small puffs of air through your mouth. Feel the air emerge over your lips. This relaxes your body and takes away your focus from leakage. It also maintains your pelvic floor muscles at an optimum tension—not too relaxed to cause leakage and not too contracted to cause fatigue.

- Pad-Free Time

This week we continue the pad-free time with the slight modification to retrain your body so you understand how much tension in your pelvic floor is necessary to avoid leaking. You will need a wide mouthed jar, such as an empty peanut butter jar, or a small bucket before you begin this exercise.

After you perform your first set of morning exercises, remove your pad or other form of leakage protection. Then, while you are sitting down as per your normal routine—for example, working on your computer or watching TV—do the following:

  −Place a plastic bag, such as a garbage bag, on your seat and cover it with a hand towel or small square disposable mattress pad if you would prefer.

  −Sit down wearing only your underwear. These will gradually become soaked, often within 30 minutes, but do not be alarmed. The reason this happens is that you have become used to the protection of the pad, and your mind does not notice or care as much about a damp pad but certainly feels the effect of wet underwear.

    a. An analogy would be getting in the habit of lifting a full bucket of water each day until your body learns to expect

the weight of the full bucket. Then one day the bucket is only half-full but you lift it with the usual amount of force, surprising you when the water spills.

–Before you stand up you will do two things: (1) place the jar under your penis so that if you leak it is caught in the container, and (2) do a Kegel while pulling in your belly. Now when you stand up you will leak immediately if you are either holding your belly and pelvic floor too tight or not tight enough. This position allows you to play around with the tension in your abdomen and pelvic floor to minimize the leak.

–The first time you do this, take two steps before you release the tension. The next day take three steps, and so forth until you reach week five. So say you take 2 steps on Monday and 3 steps on Tuesday, by that Sunday you should take 8 steps before letting go. Eventually, you should be able to make it all the way to the restroom without leaking.

–The purpose of this exercise is to get your mind and body used to returning to a pad-free lifestyle. Consistency is an important part success, but dependency needs to be avoided.

• Pad Protocol

–Use "Ultrathin" pads (heavy, medium or thin) so they will fit comfortably in your underwear.

–Make sure that the pads are "Ultrathin" so they will fit comfortably in your underwear.

–To wear, remove the sticky tape from under the pad and place inside of your Jockey underwear. Make sure that the underwear is not too tight when you put it on because the resulting discomfort may cause you to leak more.

−You will likely be changing your protective pads and Depends multiple times each day. Change them when they are soaked (generally 80% or more saturated) for consistency sake, and remember to keep track of how many you're using in the bladder log.

−Note: if your pad is too narrow and doesn't cover the base of your underwear, feel free to double up on them. You may go through them faster, but the eventual goal is to get you to be pad-free so you'll be saving in the long run—not to mention improving your quality of life—by doubling down and sticking to the regimen.

• Home Pad Use

−Continue sleeping without pads because you should not be leaking overnight at this point.

−In the morning you can begin using pantyliners. Unfortunately, my patients have not found better options for men, so pantyliners have to do. There are also many different brands available for these.

−During the rest of the day at home you can use ultrathin light absorbency pads (1 dot).

• Outside Pad Use

−Similar to last week, there is a distinction between short trips to the store, post office, neighbor's house, etc. and longer trips that require you to be out for longer than an hour. Your leak protection strategy will differ depending on which type of trip you are taking.

−On quick trips you can continue using ultrathin light absorbency pads (1 dot). These trips can be a little longer than those last week, up to two hours—for example, to pick up milk from the local grocer or mail a letter at the post office.

−On longer trips, such as shopping at the mall or socializing at a party, you should be using slightly heavier pads (2 dots). Fortunately, in America we are never too far away from the porcelain throne, and so you can almost always change your pad in a restroom if you leaked. Remember to take along extra pads, and make sure to change the one you are wearing if it gets more than half-soaked.

Exercise Protocol

•Important Points

−Do not do more than eight (8) sets of Kegels each day. A set involves 10 repetitions.

−Within reason and until you are dry avoid BLT: bending, lifting, or twisting. Repetitive BLT movements while you are trying to recover your continence post-surgery may negatively influence the coordination and contractility of the pelvic floor muscles and sphincter. In addition, intra-abdominal pressure increases when we bend, lift, or twist and the pelvic floor muscles are not yet strong enough to counteract this.

−Try not to lift anything more than 8-10 pounds in weight. That means laying off heavy housework, including but not limited to scrubbing, mopping with a cloth mop, vacuuming with a cleaner that is not self-propelled, cleaning the garage, polishing the car, remodeling the bathroom, and picking weeds. Note that this is **not a permanent** prescription, which your spouse may be happy to know!

−Do not perform abdominal, endurance, and free weight exercises while recovering this week. The only acceptable form of exercise is walking at a slow pace.

−You can do some BLT such as putting your shoes and pants on, feeding your pet, and taking clothes out of the washer/dryer.

• Kegels

−Note that the Kegel protocol changes slightly each week so it will be important for you to follow the specific steps below while keeping in mind the general form of the exercises as described in an earlier chapter.

−The first step before performing your Kegels is to update your bladder log. Remember that this should become a daily habit so that you keep track of your progress over time.

−This week we continue drawing a distinction between the complete Kegel, which involves tightening both your bottom (shutter/elevator) and your frontal (stop urinating mid-stream) pelvic floor muscles. You will still complete 8 sets, but instead of alternating between sets of complete and frontal you will do complete Kegels during sets one and eight and frontal Kegels during sets two, three, four, five, six, and seven.

−Thus, if you begin your Kegels at 6 am, an example schedule would be as follows:

- 6 am - set of *complete* Kegels with cough Kegel

- 8 am - set of frontal Kegel with cough Kegel

- 10 am - set of frontal Kegels with cough Kegel

- 12 pm - set of frontal Kegel with cough Kegel

- 2 pm - set of frontal Kegel with cough Kegel

- 4 pm - set of frontal Kegel with cough Kegel

- 6 pm - set of frontal Kegel with cough Kegel

- 8 pm - set of *complete* Kegels with cough Kegel

–Let's begin:

1. Performing a complete Kegel:

–Sit in a comfortable chair, recliner, or sofa

–Allow your mind to focus on your pelvic floor muscles.

–Begin squeezing your bottom with your muscles. One of my patients, a photographer, thought of an analogy that many of my patients find helpful. Think of your rectum like the shutter of a camera. Simply close the shutter with your mind.

–Next imagine that your closed rectum is an elevator (another analogy). Quickly raise the elevator up towards your stomach.

–While you are holding in the next step, you will simultaneously tighten your penis and scrotum by imagining that you are trying to prevent yourself from urinating. Thus, your entire pelvic region will be tightened for the count.

– **Hold for a quick count of five** (think "one, two, three, four, five," and NOT "one-Mississippi..."). Now bring it back down.

–Allow your bottom to relax completely.

–Repeat **at most** 10 times in quick succession. It should take you about 45-60 seconds, which means one second to raise the elevator, five quick-holding counts, and one second to lower it.

2. Performing a frontal Kegel

–The frontal Kegel is faster because it only involves tightening the frontal pelvic floor muscles. You can do this by imagining that you are stopping urination mid-stream.

–You should do these quickly and be able to complete 10 repetitions within 20 seconds.

3. The additional cough-Kegel

We continue the cough-Kegel at the end of each set of Kegels as described above. Here's a reminder on how to do it:

–Perform the Kegel while holding in your belly.

–During the quick-holding step, produce an artificial cough. The reason for this is to get your body used to transient increases in intra-abdominal pressure, as coughing or sneezing does. These are times when you're more likely to leak, so we are intentionally simulating it to help you overcome this problem.

–Note that this means you will be doing 8 extra cough-Kegels because they are done after each set throughout the day. Your total number of Kegels is up to 88 (80 holding Kegels and 8 cough-Kegels after each of 8 sets).

• Breathing and Other Exercises

This week you will continue two sets of the following exercises, once in the morning and once in the evening. Each set should still be 15 repetitions. Since you're becoming stronger, we'll add an additional exercise this week: the pillow squeeze.

1. First begin with a set of deep breathing exercises:

   –Breathe in through your nose and out through your mouth.

   –Your exhale should be at least twice as long as your inhale; thus, if you breathe in for 3 seconds, breathe out for 6 seconds.

   –Repeat the above 15 times total to complete the set.

   –Make sure you do not become lightheaded when doing these exercises; if you do, you are doing too many.

2. Next move on to the set of leg rolls:

   –Lie down on your back with your legs straight and spread apart by about 12 inches.

   –Inhale slowly and roll both legs inward. At the same time gently squeeze your bottom and hold for a quick count of five.

   –Now exhale, roll both legs outward, and relax your bottom.

   –Repeat the above 15 times total to complete the set.

3. The third exercise is the ball squeeze:

A few notes: It's most comfortable to do this exercise on a bed. You will need a soft, rubber ball. I highly recommend the cheap (usually under $2) 9-inch diameter balls at Walmart. Other balls, such as a football or basketball, are too sturdy.

   –Lie down on your back with your knees bent and pointed upwards and feet flat on the bed.

   –Place the ball between your knees.

–Inhale slowly while squeezing the ball and simultaneously squeezing your bottom (remember the elevator traveling towards your belly) for a quick count of five.

–Release and repeat for a total of 15 times to complete the set.

4. The fourth exercise is basically the opposite of the ball squeeze, and instead of adducting your legs you will be *abducting* them (moving them farther apart).

–Lie down on your back with your knees bent and pointed upwards and feet flat on the bed. Your legs can be close together at the starting position.

–Place the stretch band around both thighs, about 3 inches above your knees.

–Slowly move your knees apart about 8-10 inches, against the increasing tension in the band. Hold for a quick count of five.

–Repeat this 15 times.

5. The fifth exercise is the reverse abdominal.

–Lie on your back and bend both of your knees. Place your hands around one of your knees.

–Now lift that leg up so that your thigh is 90 degrees to the surface you're lying on and your knee is perpendicular to your thigh. Then bring the knee to your chest, while your hands gently push back to provide resistance. Hold for a quick count of five.

–Complete 5 repetitions to finish the set before switching over to the other leg and doing the same. Remember to do two sets each day: morning and evening.

6. The sixth exercise is the leg lift. This also works out your abdominals. This exercise and the one above are preferable to crunches because crunches increase the abdominal pressure more significantly, potentially leading to increased leaking.

–Lie on your back with one leg bent and the other straightened on the surface.

–Raise the straight leg up to about 70 degrees. Hold it for a quick count of five then bring it down.

–Complete five repetitions to finish the set before switching over to the other leg and doing the same. Remember to do two sets each day: morning and evening.

7. The seventh exercise, also targeting the abdominals, is the feet lift.

–Similar to the exercises above, lie flat on your back with both legs bent and your feet flat on the surface.

–Lift **both** feet simultaneously so that your thighs are perpendicular to the surface and your lower legs are parallel to it.

–Hold for a quick count of five, and repeat five times total to complete the set.

8. The eighth exercise is the pillow squeeze.

–Lie flat on your back with both legs bent and your feet flat on the surface.

–Place a normal-sized pillow (e.g. width is about six inches) between your knees. Squeeze for five seconds and release.

–Repeat this exercise 10 times to complete a set. As with the others, complete two sets.

9. The restroom exercise. If you want to recover even sooner, here's a secret exercise that you can incorporate into your restroom breaks.

–After you're finished on the toilet, sit with your back straight, count to 30 seconds, then lean forward and push like you are releasing gas. Repeat for a total of two times.

–The point of this is to "double-void" and empty the bladder out completely, so there is no residual urine left. This gets your body in the habit of complete emptying, which is important to prevent leakage and accidents after standing up.

10. Before doing any of the activities below follow these procedures:

For bending: do a Kegel, pull in your belly at the same time and then bend.

For lifting: Do a Kegel, at the same time pull in your belly and then lift.

For Reaching: Do a Kegel and pull in your belly at the same time and then reach for anything.

For Turning: Do a Kegel and pull in your belly at the same time and then turn.

11. If you are up and about for a long time (more than an hour), for example, golfing, shopping, walking, every 30 minutes or so gently push your rectum out for a quick count of 3, as if you are eliminating gas (flatulence). This will force your pelvic floor to relax and regroup so it can tighten and prevent leakage.

12: If you are up for more than an hour or two, remember to sit for 5 minutes and keep your feet elevated, as if you are sitting with your feet on the coffee table. This will also relax your pelvic muscle and let it regroup.

Expected Progress

After week seven you should notice the following signs of progress:

–By now going to the bathroom early in the morning should be automatic and effortless. You don't need to grab the penis or have a jar. You should be getting a strong sensation to urinate in the night and also a mild sensation in the day.

–You should be dry in the morning, meaning no pads at all during that time.

–During your trips outdoors you should be fine with one-dot pads for short distances and two-dot pads for longer periods of time.

–You should be able to restart your normal activities, such as golf, shopping, and housework.

• Take Home Points

I want to end this chapter in the same way that it began: with important points that deserve repetition because they are crucial to your recovery. Let us begin:

–Do not do Kegel exercises constantly; in fact, do not do more than 8 sets of 10 repetitions each day. Remember that the pelvic floor muscles are small, like the muscles of the hand or face, and thus, they fatigue quickly. When they are fatigued they cannot contract tightly, and when they cannot contract you leak more. **The more exercise you do past a certain point,**

the more you will leak! This sounds opposite to what society teaches us: "No pain no gain."

–When you are sitting or walking make sure that you relax your rectum and perineal areas. My patients who worry about leaking often sit with them clenched, and thus, fatigue their pelvic floor muscles, leading to more leaking. The worry about leaking becomes a self-fulfilling prophecy!

Do not try to stop the leakage right away; however, feel free to maintain a small amount of tension in your pelvic floor muscles. No matter what you do there will be at least some dribbling. It will stop. Give it time. It is a muscle. It takes at least 6-8 weeks to notice any changes after exercising other muscles, such as your abdominals or biceps, so remember that the same applies to your pelvic floor muscles. These muscles and the bladder will not strengthen and coordinate in a week!

That concludes the seventh week on your journey back to normalcy. Celebrate your accomplishments thus far and stay the course!

Chapter Fourteen

Week Eight—Getting Back to Normal

Introduction

Two more weeks to go! Let's finish strong. As always, *I will continue repeating the most important points in each chapter to make sure they are truly driven home.* Exercises require proper form, and diet should be closely followed to see the best results. These should be performed each day of the week for best results.

Must-Follow Advice

Exercise and Muscles

- **At most** do eight (8) sets of Kegels each day.

  –DO NOT DO MORE. Doing more will fatigue your pelvic floor muscles, which then will not be able to contract leading to you leaking more.

- Remember to **pull in your belly**.

The reason we pull in the abdomen (belly) is that the intra-abdominal pressure decreases. Also, if an ultrasound of the bladder is done when we pull in the belly, we are able to observe the bladder neck becoming slender, and therefore, the pelvic floor muscles—though weak—are able to tighten around the neck.

  –Before standing up. Once you are up, let your belly relax gently, but do not let go completely so you do not leak too much. You may feel a dribble, which is perfectly normal at this stage. If you forget to pull in your belly before standing up, sit back down and immediately stand up again, this time with the correct form.

–Before sitting down. Once you are seated, relax gently.

Before bending down. For example, to wipe your feet after a shower, pick something up from the floor, or put your shoes on.

- When sitting make sure your **bottom is relaxed**.

  –If you sit with your bottom squeezed tightly, you will eventually feel pain in your rectal and genital areas. This will lead to increased leakage, again due to muscle fatigue.

  –This is one reason deep breathing is such an important exercise. Breathe in through your lips, then as you breathe out, relax your bottom.

- When standing make sure your **bottom is relaxed**.

  –Whenever you are standing for extended periods of time—for example, waiting in line at the grocery store—make sure that your rectal and genital area is relaxed. People tend to constantly be clenching because they are afraid to leak.

  –The best way I've found for having my patients relax is to have them pretend to pass gas for a quick count of three, which will then help them relax their bottom and overall decrease muscle fatigue.

- **Breathe** on your way to the restroom.

  –On your way to the restroom, blow small puffs of air through your mouth. Feel the air emerge over your lips. This relaxes your body and takes away your focus from leakage. It also maintains your pelvic floor muscles at an optimum tension— not too relaxed to cause leakage and not too contracted to cause fatigue.

• Pad-Free Time

This week we continue the pad-free time with the slight modification to retrain your body so you understand how much tension in your pelvic floor is necessary to avoid leaking. You will need a wide mouthed jar, such as an empty peanut butter jar, or a small bucket before you begin this exercise.

After you perform your first set of morning exercises, remove your pad or other form of leakage protection. Then, while you are sitting down as per your normal routine—for example working on your computer or watching TV—do the following:

–Place a plastic bag, such as a garbage bag, on your seat and cover it with a hand towel or small square disposable mattress pad if you would prefer.

–Sit down wearing only your underwear. These will gradually become soaked, often within 30 minutes, but do not be alarmed. The reason this happens is that you have become used to the protection of the pad, and your mind does not notice or care as much about a damp pad but certainly feels the effect of wet underwear.

a. An analogy would be getting in the habit of lifting a full bucket of water each day until your body learns to expect the weight of the full bucket. Then one day the bucket is only half-full but you lift it with the usual amount of force, surprising you when the water spills.

165

–Before you stand up you will do two things: (1) place the jar under your penis so that if you leak it is caught in the container, and (2) do a Kegel while pulling in your belly. Now when you stand up you will leak immediately if you are either holding your belly and pelvic floor too tight or not tight enough. This position allows you to play around with the tension in your abdomen and pelvic floor to minimize the leak.

–The first time you do this, take two steps before you release the tension. The next day take three steps, and so forth until you reach week five. So say you take 2 steps on Monday and 3 steps on Tuesday, by that Sunday you should take 8 steps before letting go. Eventually you should be able to make it all the way to the restroom without leaking.

–The purpose of this exercise is to get your mind and body used to returning to a pad-free lifestyle. Consistency is an important part success, but dependency needs to be avoided.

• Pad Protocol

–Use "Ultrathin" pads (heavy, medium or thin) so they will fit comfortably in your underwear.

–Make sure that the pads are "Ultrathin" so they will fit comfortably in your underwear.

–To wear, remove the sticky tape from under the pad and place inside of your Jockey underwear. Make sure that the underwear is not too tight when you put it on because the resulting discomfort may cause you to leak more.

–You will likely be changing your protective pads and Depends multiple times each day. Change them when they are soaked (generally 80% or more saturated) for consistency sake, and remember to keep track of how many you're using in the bladder log.

−Note: if your pad is too narrow and doesn't cover the base of your underwear, feel free to double up on them. You may go through them faster, but the eventual goal is to get you to be pad-free so you'll be saving in the long run—not to mention improving your quality of life—by doubling down and sticking to the regimen.

• Home Pad Use

   −Just like last week, continue refraining from pads while you sleep.

   −In the morning use pantyliners. Unfortunately, my patients have not found better options for men, so pantyliners have to do. There are also many different brands available for these.

   −During the rest of the day at home you should be minimizing your use of ultrathin light absorbency pads (1 dot).

• Outside Pad Use

   −This week you should begin using the ultrathin light absorbency pads (1 dot) for all trips that you take outside, long or short. We continue to step down the amount of protection you need, physically and psychologically.

   −Fortunately, in America we are never too far away from the porcelain throne, and so you can almost always change your pad in a restroom if you leaked. Remember to take along extra pads, and make sure to change the one you are wearing if it gets more than half-soaked.

- Exercise Protocol

Important Points:

–Do not do more than eight (8) sets of Kegels each day. A set involves 10 repetitions.

–Within reason and until you are dry avoid BLT: bending, lifting, or twisting. Repetitive BLT movements while you are trying to recover your continence post-surgery may negatively influence the coordination and contractility of the pelvic floor muscles and sphincter. In addition, intra-abdominal pressure increases when we bend, lift, or twist and the pelvic floor muscles are not yet strong enough to counteract this.

–Try not to lift anything more than 8-10 pounds in weight. That means laying off heavy housework, including but not limited to scrubbing, mopping with a cloth mop, vacuuming with a cleaner that is not self-propelled, cleaning the garage, polishing the car, remodeling the bathroom, and picking weeds. Note that this is **not a permanent** prescription, which your spouse may be happy to know!

–Do not perform abdominal, endurance, and free weight exercises while recovering this week. The only acceptable form of exercise is walking at a slow pace.

–You can do some BLT such as putting your shoes and pants on, feeding your pet, and taking clothes out of the washer/dryer.

- Kegels

–Note that the Kegel protocol changes slightly each week so it will be important for you to follow the specific steps below while keeping in mind the general form of the exercises as described in an earlier chapter.

The first step before performing your Kegels is to update your bladder log. Remember that this should become a daily habit so that you keep track of your progress over time.

This week we continue drawing a distinction between the complete Kegel, which involves tightening both your bottom (shutter/elevator) and your frontal (stop urinating mid-stream) pelvic floor muscles. The only difference is that instead of doing the frontal Kegels in the span of 20 seconds, you can do them slower (30 seconds) to build up endurance.

Thus, if you begin your Kegels at 6 am, an example schedule would be as follows:

- 6 am - set of *complete* Kegels with cough Kegel

- 8 am - set of frontal Kegel with cough Kegel

- 10 am - set of frontal Kegels with cough Kegel

- 12 pm - set of frontal Kegel with cough Kegel

- 2 pm - set of frontal Kegel with cough Kegel

- 4 pm - set of frontal Kegel with cough Kegel

- 6 pm - set of frontal Kegel with cough Kegel

- 8 pm - set of *complete* Kegels with cough Kegel

–Let's begin:

1. Performing a complete Kegel:

–Sit in a comfortable chair, recliner, or sofa

−Allow your mind to focus on your pelvic floor muscles.

−Begin squeezing your bottom with your muscles. One of my patients, a photographer, thought of an analogy that many of my patients find helpful. Think of your rectum like the shutter of a camera. Simply close the shutter with your mind.

−Next imagine that your closed rectum is an elevator (another analogy). Quickly raise the elevator up towards your stomach.

−While you are holding in the next step, you will simultaneously tighten your penis and scrotum by imagining that you are trying to prevent yourself from urinating. Thus, your entire pelvic region will be tightened for the count.

−**Hold for a quick count of five** (think "one, two, three, four, five," and NOT "one-Mississippi..."). Now bring it back down.

−Allow your bottom to relax completely.

−Repeat **at most** 10 times in quick succession. It should take you about 45-60 seconds, which means one second to raise the elevator, five quick-holding counts, and one second to lower it.

2. Performing a frontal Kegel in week 8

The frontal Kegel is faster because it only involves tightening the frontal pelvic floor muscles. You can do this by imagining that you are stopping urination mid-stream.

−This week you should go a little slower than you are used to: complete 10 repetitions in around 30 seconds, as opposed to 20 seconds.

3. **The additional cough-Kegel**. We continue the cough-Kegel at the end of each set of Kegels as described above. Here's a reminder on how to do it:

—Perform the Kegel while holding in your belly.

—During the quick-holding step, produce an artificial cough. The reason for this is to get your body used to transient increases in intra-abdominal pressure, as coughing or sneezing does. These are times when you're more likely to leak, so we are intentionally simulating it to help you overcome this problem.

—Note that this means you will be doing 8 extra cough-Kegels because they are done after each set throughout the day. Your total number of Kegels is up to 88 (80 holding Kegels and 8 cough-Kegels after each of 8 sets).

• Breathing and Other Exercises

This week you will continue two sets of the following exercises, once in the morning and once in the evening. Each set should be 20 repetitions unless otherwise stated. Since you're becoming stronger, this week there is another exercise: the mini squat!

1. First begin with a set of deep breathing exercises:

—Breathe in through your nose and out through your mouth.

—Your exhale should be at least twice as long as your inhale; thus, if you breathe in for 3 seconds, breathe out for 6 seconds.

—Repeat the above 20 times total to complete the set.

—Make sure you do not become lightheaded when doing these exercises; if you do, you are doing too many.

2. Next move on to the set of leg rolls:

–Lie down on your back with your legs straight and spread apart by about 12 inches.

–Inhale slowly and roll both legs inward. At the same time gently squeeze your bottom and hold for a quick count of five.

–Now exhale, roll both legs outward, and relax your bottom.

–Repeat the above 20 times total to complete the set.

3. The third exercise is the ball squeeze:

A few notes: It's most comfortable to do this exercise on a bed. You will need a soft, rubber ball. I highly recommend the cheap (usually under $2) 9-inch diameter balls at Walmart. Other balls, such as a football or basketball, are too sturdy.

–Lie down on your back with your knees bent and pointed upwards and feet flat on the bed.

–Place the ball between your knees.

–Inhale slowly while squeezing the ball and simultaneously squeezing your bottom (remember the elevator traveling towards your belly) for a quick count of five.

–Release and repeat for a total of 20 times to complete the set.

4. The fourth exercise is basically the opposite of the ball squeeze and instead of adducting your legs you will be *abducting* them (moving them farther apart).

–Lie down on your back with your knees bent and pointed upwards and feet flat on the bed. Your legs can be close together at the starting position.

–Place the stretch band around both thighs, about 3 inches above your knees.

–Slowly move your knees apart about 8-10 inches, against the increasing tension in the band. Hold for a quick count of five.

–Repeat this 20 times.

5. The fifth exercise is the reverse abdominal.

–Lie on your back and bend both of your knees. Place your hands around one of your knees.

–Now lift that leg up so that your thigh is 90 degrees to the surface you're lying on and your knee is perpendicular to your thigh. Then bring the knee to your chest, while your hands gently push back to provide resistance. Hold for a quick count of five.

–Complete 10 repetitions to finish the set before switching over to the other leg and doing the same. Remember to do two sets each day: morning and evening.

6. The sixth exercise is the leg lift.

This also works out your abdominals. This exercise and the one above are preferable to crunches because crunches increase the abdominal pressure more significantly, potentially leading to increased leaking.

–Lie on your back with one leg bent and the other straightened on the surface.

–Raise the straight leg up to about 70 degrees. Hold it for a quick count of five then bring it down.

–Complete 10 repetitions to finish the set before switching over to the other leg and doing the same. Remember to do two sets each day: morning and evening.

7. The seventh exercise, also targeting the abdominals, is the feet lift.

–Similar to the exercises above, lie flat on your back with both legs bent and your feet flat on the surface.

–Lift **both** feet simultaneously so that your thighs are perpendicular to the surface and your lower legs are parallel to it.

–Hold for a quick count of five, and repeat 10 times total to complete the set. Do two sets each day: morning and evening.

8. The eighth exercise is the pillow squeeze.

–Lie flat on your back with both legs bent and your feet flat on the surface.

–Place a normal-sized pillow (e.g. width is about six inches) between your knees. Squeeze for five seconds and release.

–Repeat this exercise 10 times to complete a set. As with the others, complete two sets.

9. The ninth exercise is the mini squat.

–Stand behind a chair, grasping the top bar firmly. Keep your feet shoulder-width apart.

–Inhale while doing a full Kegel, pulling in your belly, and squatting part-way. Do not go all the way down where your thighs are parallel to the ground, instead do a mini squat.

Now exhale while standing up and relaxing your pelvic floor muscles.

Repeat this exercise 10 times to complete a set. As with the other exercises, complete two sets.

10. **The restroom exercise.** If you want to recover even sooner, here's a secret exercise that you can incorporate into your restroom breaks.

–After you're finished on the toilet, sit with your back straight, count to 30 seconds, then lean forward and push like you are releasing gas. Repeat for a total of two times.

–The point of this is to "double-void" and empty the bladder out completely, so there is no residual urine left. This gets your body in the habit of complete emptying, which is important to prevent leakage and accidents after standing up.

11. Before doing any of the activities below follow these procedures:

For bending: do a Kegel, pull in your belly at the same time and then bend.

For lifting: Do a Kegel, at the same time pull in your belly and then lift.

For Reaching: Do a Kegel and pull in your belly at the same time and then reach for anything.

For Turning: Do a Kegel and pull in your belly at the same time and then turn.

12. If you are up and about for a long time (more than an hour), for example, golfing, shopping, walking, every 30 minutes or so gently push your rectum out for a quick count of 3, as if you are eliminating gas (flatulence). This will force your pelvic floor to relax and regroup so it can tighten and prevent leakage.

13: If you are up for more than an hour or two, remember to sit for 5 minutes and keep your feet elevated, as if you are sitting with your feet on the coffee table. This will also relax your pelvic muscle and let it regroup.

Expected progress

After week 8 you should be completely pad free inside of the house and require fewer pads during your trips outside of the house (all should be one-dot). You can continue returning to normal activities.

• Take Home Points

I want to end this chapter in the same way that it began: with important points that deserve repetition because they are crucial to your recovery. Let us begin:

–Do not do Kegel exercises constantly; in fact, do not do more than 8 sets of 10 repetitions each day. Remember that the pelvic floor muscles are small, like the muscles of the hand or face, and thus, they fatigue quickly. When they are fatigued they cannot contract tightly, and when they cannot contract you leak more. **The more exercise you do past a certain point, the more you will leak!** This sounds opposite to what society teaches us: "No pain no gain."

–When you are sitting or walking make sure that you relax your rectum and perineal areas. My patients who worry about leaking often sit with them clenched, and thus, fatigue their pelvic floor muscles, leading to more leaking. The worry about leaking becomes a self-fulfilling prophecy!

–Do not try to stop the leakage right away; however, feel free to maintain a small amount of tension in your pelvic floor muscles. No matter what you do there will be at least some dribbling. It will stop. Give it time. It is a muscle. It takes at least 6-8 weeks to notice any changes after exercising other muscles, such as your abdominals or biceps, so remember that the same applies to your pelvic floor muscles. These muscles and the bladder will not strengthen and coordinate in a week!

That concludes the eight week on your journey back to normalcy. Celebrate your accomplishments thus far and stay the course!

Chapter Fifteen

Week Nine—Made It!

Introduction

You've made it! This is the last week of the program. By now you should we well on your way to an active and pad-free lifestyle.

As always, *I will continue repeating the most important points in each chapter to make sure they are truly driven home*. Exercises require proper form, and diet should be closely followed to see the best results. These should be performed each day of the week for best results.

Must-Follow Advice

Exercise and Muscles

- **At most** do eight (8) sets of Kegels each day.

    –DO NOT DO MORE. Doing more will fatigue your pelvic floor muscles, which then will not be able to contract leading to you leaking more.

- Remember to **pull in your belly**.

The reason we pull in the abdomen (belly) is that the intra-abdominal pressure decreases. Also, if an ultrasound of the bladder is done when we pull in the belly, we are able to observe the bladder neck becoming slender, and therefore, the pelvic floor muscles—though weak—are able to tighten around the neck.

–Before standing up. Once you are up, let your belly relax gently, but do not let go completely so you do not leak too much. You may feel a dribble, which is perfectly normal at this stage. If you forget to pull in your belly before standing up, sit back down and immediately stand up again, this time with the correct form.

–Before sitting down. Once you are seated, relax gently.

–Before bending down. For example, to wipe your feet after a shower, pick something up from the floor, or put your shoes on.

• When sitting make sure your **bottom is relaxed**.

–If you sit with your bottom squeezed tightly, you will eventually feel pain in your rectal and genital areas. This will lead to increased leakage, again due to muscle fatigue.

–This is one reason deep breathing is such an important exercise. Breathe in through your lips, then as you breathe out, relax your bottom.

• When standing make sure your **bottom is relaxed**.

–Whenever you are standing for extended periods of time—for example by waiting in line at the grocery store—make sure that your rectal and genital area is relaxed. People tend to constantly be clenching because they are afraid to leak.

–The best way I've found for having my patients relax is to have them pretend to pass gas for a quick count of three, which will then help them relax their bottom and overall decrease muscle fatigue.

- **Breathe** on your way to the restroom.

    –On your way to the restroom, blow small puffs of air through your mouth. Feel the air emerge over your lips. This relaxes your body and takes away your focus from leakage. It also maintains your pelvic floor muscles at an optimum tension; not too relaxed to cause leakage and not too contracted to cause fatigue.

- Pad-Free Time

This week we continue the pad-free time with the slight modification to retrain your body so you understand how much tension in your pelvic floor is necessary to avoid leaking. You will need a wide mouthed jar, such as an empty peanut butter jar, or a small bucket before you begin this exercise.

After you perform your first set of morning exercises, remove your pad or other form of leakage protection. Then, while you are sitting down as per your normal routine—for example working on your computer or watching TV—do the following:

    –Place a plastic bag, such as a garbage bag, on your seat and cover it with a hand towel or small square disposable mattress pad if you would prefer.

    –Sit down wearing only your jockey shorts or underwear. These will gradually become soaked, often within 10 minutes, but do not be alarmed. The reason this happens is that you have become used to the protection of the pad, and your mind does not notice or care as much about a damp pad but certainly feels the effect of wet underwear.

    a. An analogy would be getting in the habit of lifting a full bucket of water each day until your body learns to expect

the weight of the full bucket. Then one day the bucket is only half-full but you lift it with the usual amount of force, surprising you when the water spills.

–Before you stand up you will do two things: (1) place the jar under your penis so that if you leak it is caught in the container, and (2) do a Kegel while pulling in your belly. Now when you stand up you will leak immediately if you are either holding your belly and pelvic floor too tight or not tight enough. This position allows you to play around with the tension in your abdomen and pelvic floor to minimize the leak.

–The first time you do this, take two steps before you release the tension. The next day take three steps, and so forth until you reach week five. So say you take 2 steps on Monday and 3 steps on Tuesday, by that Sunday you should take 8 steps before letting go. Eventually, you should be able to make it all the way to the restroom without leaking.

–The purpose of this exercise is to get your mind and body used to returning to a pad-free lifestyle. Consistency is an important part success, but dependency needs to be avoided.

• Pad Protocol

–Use "Ultrathin" pads so they will fit comfortably in your underwear.

–To wear, remove the sticky tape from under the pad and place inside of your Jockey underwear. Make sure that the underwear is not too tight when you put it on because the resulting discomfort may cause you to leak more.

–You will likely be changing your protective pads and Depends multiple times each day. Change them when they are soaked (generally 80% or more saturated) for consistency sake, and remember to keep track of how many you're using in the bladder log.

–Note: if your pad is too narrow and doesn't cover the base of your underwear, feel free to double up on them. You may go through them faster, but the eventual goal is to get you to be pad-free so you'll be saving in the long run—not to mention improving your quality of life—by doubling down and sticking to the regimen.

• Home Pad Use

–Just like last week, continue refraining from pads while you sleep.

–In the morning use pantyliners. Unfortunately, my patients have not found better options for men, so pantyliners have to do. There are also many different brands available for these.

–During the rest of the day at home you should be minimizing your use of ultrathin light absorbency pads (1 dot).

• Outside Pad Use

–Continue stepping down your use of pads. While you can use ultrathin light absorbency pads (1 dot) for all trips that you take outside, long or short, try taking short trips without pad protection. We continue to step down the amount of protection you need, physically and psychologically.

–Fortunately, in America we are never too far away from the porcelain throne, and so you can almost always change your pad in a restroom if you leaked. Remember to take along extra pads, and make sure to change the one you are wearing if it gets more than half-soaked.

• Exercise Protocol

Important Points:

–Do not do more than eight (8) sets of Kegels each day. A set involves 10 repetitions.

–Within reason and until you are dry avoid BLT: bending, lifting, or twisting. Repetitive BLT movements while you are trying to recover your continence post-surgery may negatively influence the coordination and contractility of the pelvic floor muscles and sphincter. In addition, intra-abdominal pressure increases when we bend, lift, or twist and the pelvic floor muscles are not yet strong enough to counteract this.

–Try not to lift anything more than 8-10 pounds in weight. That means laying off heavy housework, including but not limited to scrubbing, mopping with a cloth mop, vacuuming with a cleaner that is not self-propelled, cleaning the garage, polishing the car, remodeling the bathroom, and picking weeds. Note that this is **not a permanent** prescription, which your spouse may be happy to know!

–Do not perform abdominal, endurance, and free weight exercises while recovering this week. The only acceptable form of exercise is walking at a slow pace.

–You can do some BLT such as putting your shoes and pants on, feeding your pet, and taking clothes out of the washer/dryer.

• Kegels

Note that the Kegel protocol changes slightly each week so it will be important for you to follow the specific steps below while keeping in mind the general form of the exercises as described in an earlier chapter.

The first step before performing your Kegels is to update your bladder log. Remember that this should become a daily habit so that you keep track of your progress over time.

This week we continue drawing a distinction between the complete Kegel, which involves tightening both your bottom (shutter/elevator) and your frontal (stop urinating mid-stream) pelvic floor muscles. This week you will continue doing frontal Kegels at the slower pace of 30 seconds, and instead of doing complete Kegels with a quick count of five, you'll hold for a quick count of seven.

–Thus, if you begin your Kegels at 6 am, an example schedule would be as follows:

- 6 am - set of *complete* Kegels with cough Kegel

- 8 am - set of frontal Kegel with cough Kegel

- 10 am - set of frontal Kegels with cough Kegel

- 12 pm - set of frontal Kegel with cough Kegel

- 2 pm - set of frontal Kegel with cough Kegel

- 4 pm - set of frontal Kegel with cough Kegel

- 6 pm - set of frontal Kegel with cough Kegel

- 8 pm - set of *complete* Kegels with cough Kegel

–Let's begin:

185

1. Performing a complete Kegel:

–Sit in a comfortable chair, recliner, or sofa

–Allow your mind to focus on your pelvic floor muscles.

–Begin squeezing your bottom with your muscles. One of my patients, a photographer, thought of an analogy that many of my patients find helpful. Think of your rectum like the shutter of a camera. Simply close the shutter with your mind.

–Next imagine that your closed rectum is an elevator (another analogy). Quickly raise the elevator up towards your stomach.

–While you are holding in the next step, you will simultaneously tighten your penis and scrotum by imagining that you are trying to prevent yourself from urinating. Thus, your entire pelvic region will be tightened for the count.

–**Hold for a quick count of seven** (think "one, two, three, four, five, six, seven" and NOT "one-Mississippi…"). Now bring it back down.

–Allow your bottom to relax completely.

–Repeat **at most** 10 times in quick succession. It should take you about 45-60 seconds, which means one second to raise the elevator, five quick holding counts, and one second to lower it.

2. Performing a frontal Kegel in week 8

–The frontal Kegel is faster because it only involves tightening the frontal pelvic floor muscles. You can do this by imagining that you are stopping urination mid-stream.

−This week you should go a little slower than you are used to: complete 10 repetitions in around 30 seconds, as opposed to 20 seconds.

3. **The additional cough-Kegel.** We continue the cough-Kegel at the end of each set of Kegels as described above. Here's a reminder on how to do it:

−Perform the Kegel while holding in your belly.

−During the quick-holding step produce an artificial cough. The reason for this is to get your body used to transient increases in intra-abdominal pressure, as coughing or sneezing does. These are times when you're more likely to leak, so we are intentionally simulating it to help you overcome this problem.

−Note that this means you will be doing 8 extra cough-Kegels because they are done after each set throughout the day. Your total number of Kegels is up to 88 (80 holding Kegels and 8 cough-Kegels after each of 8 sets).

• Breathing and Other Exercises

This week you will continue two sets of the following exercises, once in the morning and once in the evening. Each set should still be 20 repetitions unless otherwise stated. And don't worry, this week we aren't adding another exercise! Should be a cinch to do.

1. First begin with a set of deep breathing exercises:

−Breathe in through your nose and out through your mouth.

−Your exhale should be at least twice as long as your inhale; thus, if you breathe in for 3 seconds, breathe out for 6 seconds.

–Repeat the above 20 times total to complete the set.

–Make sure you do not become lightheaded when doing these exercises; if you do, you are doing too many.

2. Next move on to the set of leg rolls:

–Lie down on your back with your legs straight and spread apart by about 12 inches.

–Inhale slowly and roll both legs inward. At the same time gently squeeze your bottom and hold for a quick count of five.

–Now exhale, roll both legs outward, and relax your bottom.

–Repeat the above 20 times total to complete the set.

3. The third exercise is the ball squeeze:

A few notes: It's most comfortable to do this exercise on a bed. You will need a soft, rubber ball. I highly recommend the cheap (usually under $2) 9-inch diameter balls at Walmart. Other balls, such as a football or basketball, are too sturdy.

–Lie down on your back with your knees bent and pointed upwards and feet flat on the bed.

–Place the ball between your knees.

–Inhale slowly while squeezing the ball and simultaneously squeezing your bottom (remember the elevator traveling towards your belly) for a quick count of five.

–Release and repeat for a total of 20 times to complete the set.

4. The fourth exercise is basically the opposite of the ball squeeze and instead of adducting your legs you will be *abducting* them (moving them farther apart).

–Lie down on your back with your knees bent and pointed upwards and feet flat on the bed. Your legs can be close together at the starting position.

–Place the stretch band around both thighs, about 3 inches above your knees.

–Slowly move your knees apart about 8-10 inches, against the increasing tension in the band. Hold for a quick count of 5.

–Repeat this 20 times.

5. The fifth exercise is the reverse abdominal.

–Lie on your back and bend both of your knees. Place your hands around one of your knees.

–Now lift that leg up so that your thigh is 90 degrees to the surface you're lying on and your knee is perpendicular to your thigh. Then bring the knee to your chest, while your hands gently push back to provide resistance. Hold for a quick count of five.

–Complete 10 repetitions to finish the set before switching over to the other leg and doing the same. Remember to do two sets each day: morning and evening.

6. The sixth exercise is the leg lift.

This also works out your abdominals. This exercise and the one above are preferable to crunches because crunches increase the abdominal pressure more significantly, potentially leading to increased leaking.

–Lie on your back with one leg bent and the other straightened on the surface.

–Raise the straight leg up to about 70 degrees. Hold it for a quick count of five then bring it down.

–Complete 10 repetitions to finish the set before switching over to the other leg and doing the same. Remember to do two sets each day: morning and evening.

7. The seventh exercise, also targeting the abdominals, is the feet lift.

–Similar to the exercises above, lie flat on your back with both legs bent and your feet flat on the surface.

–Lift **both** feet simultaneously so that your thighs are perpendicular to the surface and your lower legs are parallel to it.

–Hold for a quick count of five, and repeat ten times total to complete the set. Do two sets each day: morning and evening.

8. The eighth exercise is the pillow squeeze.

–Lie flat on your back with both legs bent and your feet flat on the surface.

–Place a normal-sized pillow (e.g. width is about six inches) between your knees. Squeeze for five seconds and release.

–Repeat this exercise 10 times to complete a set. As with the others, complete two sets.

9. The ninth exercise is the mini squat.

–Stand behind a chair, grasping the top bar firmly. Keep your feet shoulder-width apart.

–Inhale while doing a full Kegel, pulling in your belly, and squatting part way. Do not go all the way down where your thighs are parallel to the ground; instead, do a mini squat.

–Now exhale while standing up and relaxing your pelvic floor muscles.

–Repeat this exercise 10 times to complete a set. As with the other exercises, complete two sets.

10. **The restroom exercise**. If you want to recover even sooner, here's a secret exercise that you can incorporate into your restroom breaks.

-After you're finished on the toilet, sit with your back straight, count to 30 seconds, then lean forward and push like you are releasing gas. Repeat for a total of two times.

-The point of this is to "double-void" and empty the bladder out completely, so there is no residual urine left. This gets your body in the habit of complete emptying, which is important to prevent leakage and accidents after standing up.

11. Before doing any of the activities below follow these procedures:

For bending: do a Kegel, pull in your belly at the same time and then bend.

For lifting: Do a Kegel, at the same time pull in your belly and then lift.

For Reaching: Do a Kegel and pull in your belly at the same time and then reach for anything.

For Turning: Do a Kegel and pull in your belly at the same time and then turn.

12. If you are up and about for a long time (more than an hour), for example, golfing, shopping, walking, every 30 minutes or so gently push your rectum out for a quick count of 3, as if you are eliminating gas (flatulence). This will force your pelvic floor to relax and regroup so it can tighten and prevent leakage.

13: If you are up for more than an hour or two, remember to sit for 5 minutes and keep your feet elevated, as if you are sitting with your feet on the coffee table. This will also relax your pelvic muscle and let it regroup.

Expected Progress

At this point if all has gone well you should be back to normal! Here's what my patients report at the end of the program:

–Normal sensation to urinate, with a good stream.

–Dry all day.

–Using thin panty liners during exercise and longer trips outside of the house, just in case.

•Take Home Points

I want to end this chapter in the same way that it began: with important points that deserve repetition because they are crucial to your recovery. Let us begin:

–Do not do Kegel exercises constantly; in fact, do not do more than 8 sets of 10 repetitions each day. Remember that the pelvic floor muscles are small, like the muscles of the hand or face, and thus, they fatigue quickly. When they are fatigued they cannot contract tightly, and when they cannot contract you leak more. **The more exercise you do past a certain point, the more you will leak!** This sounds opposite to what society teaches us: "No pain no gain."

–When you are sitting or walking make sure that you relax your rectum and perineal areas. My patients who worry about leaking often sit with them clenched, and thus, fatigue their pelvic floor muscles, leading to more leaking. The worry about leaking becomes a self-fulfilling prophecy!

Do not try to stop the leakage right away; however, feel free to maintain a small amount of tension in your pelvic floor muscles. No matter what you do there will be at least some dribbling. It will stop. Give it time. It is a muscle. It takes at least 6-8 weeks to notice any changes after exercising other muscles, such as your abdominals or biceps, so remember that the same applies to your pelvic floor muscles. These muscles and the bladder will not strengthen and coordinate in a week!

Congratulations! You have finished all nine weeks. That is an accomplishment that you should be proud of. More importantly by now you should be well on your way back to a free, active lifestyle!

Chapter Sixteen

Week Ten—Back to Normal

Introduction

Y ou should now be doing everything normally, like you were prior to surgery. Remember these final points as you continue your progression toward becoming fully continent. Continue all exercises in week nine.

The **must do** protocol changes slightly.

1. Before you stand up:

a. take two deep breaths, relax your bottom (imagine you bottom is a blob which just spreads out when dropped on a flat surface).

b. Push out imaginary flatulence twice quickly for a quick count of 3 (1.2.3).

c. Perform two quick complete Kegels (1.2).

d. Pull in your belly, stand up, relax you belly and walk normally either to the kitchen, bathroom, another room or wherever you want to go.

2. DON'T ANALYZE. Don't think about holding leaking. Divert your mind towards another task—like cleaning the car, pressure washing, checking email, etc. Just get up and walk normally as though you never had surgery.

3. If you feel a couple of drops of leakage then perform two quick complete Kegels.

4. If you lift something and feel a bit of urine again, perform two quick Kegels. Make sure your buttocks, rectum, etc. are not being held tightly.

5. If you are sitting on the patio, working in the yard or going to the pool, remember to wear swimming trunks and shorts without a pad. Just forget about the surgery—put it in the back of your mind

6. The important factor now is not to obsess anymore about leaking, getting dry, just get on with your daily activities and try to forget that you had this surgery.

7. DO NOT GET TEMPTED TO WEAR LARGER PADS or you will regress.

8. Before doing any of the activities below follow these procedures:

For bending: do a Kegel, pull in your belly at the same time and then bend.
For lifting: Do a Kegel, at the same time pull in your belly and then lift.
For Reaching: Do a Kegel and pull in your belly at the same time and then reach for anything.

For Turning: Do a Kegel and pull in your belly at the same time and then turn.

9. If you are up and about for a long time (more than an hour), for example, golfing, shopping, walking, every 30 minutes or so gently push your rectum out for a quick count of 3, as if you are eliminating gas (flatulence). This will force your pelvic floor to relax and regroup so it can tighten and prevent leakage.

10. If you are up for more than an hour or two, remember to sit for 5 minutes and keep your feet elevated, as if you are sitting with your feet on the coffee table. This will also relax your pelvic muscle and let it regroup.

Enjoy the feeling of being back to normal.

Part Three:

Conclusion

Chapter Fifteen:

Trouble-Shooting

In the event that you should occasionally have these lingering incidents, here are some trouble-shooting tips:

• While standing, if you feel a little bit of urine trickling down, perform two quick front Kegels. That should stop the leakage.

• While walking, if you feel a sudden leakage, perform deep breathing and make sure your bottom is relaxed.

• Make sure you drink plenty of water—especially on days of increased activity—to avoid concentration of uric acid and bladder irritation.

• If you are dry for a period of time and then suddenly there is an increase in leakage, stop the Kegels for for a couple of days so your pelvic floor muscle can relax and recover. Sometimes when we are dry and then start leaking again the temptation to do too many Kegels or do too many exercises becomes very strong, resulting in increased leakage.

• If you take a water pill (Lasix) you will notice the leakage is more. We have found that taking your water pill (Lasix) around 4:00 AM or 5:00 AM decreases leakage.

• If there is an increase in leakage, check for these three things:

   a. You drank too much water,

   b. You did not drink enough water,

c. You ate food with too much salt, sugar, or preservatives.

• Sometimes you may get a feeling that you are leaking, but this is just a perception, because when you check your pad you'll notice it's dry.

• If you're waking up several times a night to urinate it may be due to highly concentrated urine and an irritated bladder. You can try the following suggestions, which have worked for my patients who report sleeping longer after a few days:

a. Make sure your medications are taken by 7 pm,

b. Drink an 8 oz. glass of water right before you sleep,

c. Each time you wake up drink 3 oz. of water.

• If you find that certain movements cause a sudden squirt of urine to leak out, remember to practice performing those movements while pulling in your belly and performing a Kegel at the same time. For example, if you bend down to pick up something up from the floor and leak while doing so, the next time remember to pull in your belly and perform a Kegel.

• Tight underwear or diapers are not conducive to achieving continence. Make sure that your underwear and diapers are the correct size and fit comfortably.

Conclusion

This book has taken a long time being written. It has been made possible with a lot of encouragement from my patients who felt that they would have done better if they had known what to expect. Also, they had many relatives and friends around the country who had never heard of Physical Therapy to improve bladder function.

In addition, they had read online in forums and blogs that the national average to being continent was 6 months to 2 years, and they have been really pleased that they were continent in 10 weeks. I hope this book will meet all your expectations and help you achieve continence in a short period of time.

Follow all the guidelines in this book as they have been written. Do not add your own protocol or mix and match the protocol from different websites and schools of thought or hospitals.

I would like to emphasize and reemphasize that you will not get dry in a week or a couple of weeks, even if you follow the directions in this book. Please remember that recovery time from hip, knee, elbow, or shoulder surgeries are 6-12 weeks, barring all complications. The pelvic floor muscle and the bladder are muscles, and they will take a few weeks as well.

In addition in training to be continent, we have to take three factors in account—the brain, the bladder and the pelvic floor. When all of these sync together we achieve continence. There has to be coordination of all three to become dry. This is one of the main reasons that patients first get dry during the night. They are sleeping, and the brain and bladder do what they are supposed to do. A full bladder sends the signal to the brain, which then sends a signal to the PFM, which then contracts appropriately to prevent leakage—and then you walk to the toilet and void there.

So now I leave you with this book and lots of good wishes for a complete recovery from this traumatic phase in your life. As always, if you have any individual questions or concerns feel free to email me and I will try to respond to answer your questions and concerns.

I hope by following the advice in this book you'll be able to achieve continence in the shortest period of time...

Good luck and God Bless

-Vanita Gaglani

Additional Acknowledgements

I would like to acknowledge a few people who helped make this book a reality:

Anushka Gaglani, our daughter: She jump-started my book by making sense, rewriting and putting my thoughts into words.

Shiv Gaglani, our son, who took over from his sister and made the book a reality. He worked extremely hard, organizing the content, contacting Jean (my editor and book designer), and making it perfect. This while starting two companies of his own at the same time.

Mukesh Gaglani, my husband: He patiently typed and made my forms a reality since I am so technically challenged.

Jean Boles: A wonderful editor who knew exactly where to take over from Shiv and format the book.

Ryan Bailey, who illustrated the diagrams.

Bonnie Nelson, who illustrated the pelvic floor for me.

James McKinley and his wonderful wife, Barbara, one of my favorite patients and his wife, who kept calling me to see if I had started the book.

Joseph Alenski and his wonderful wife, another favorite patient.

Derek. E: His greatest compliment was telling his friends and other patients "If Vanita says stand on one leg, do it; don't question it, just do it."

Donald M: He made the bladder logs on Excel and modified and re-modified them multiple times to where every patient's input was added.

All my other patients who fondly say to me, "We love you but don't take it personally if we never want to see you again." They do pop in to say a hello in spite of that.

ustoo.org: I learned a lot from them about other issues including erectile dysfunction, and emotional problems that are associated with prostate cancer.

Recommended Books and Websites

1. Dr. Patrick Walsh's *Guide To Surviving Prostate Cancer*

2. Strum, Stephen and Pagliano, Donna

3. Mulhall, John: *Saving Your Sex Life: A Guide For Men With Prostate Cancer*

4. Howard Clark: www.clarkhoward.com

5. Blum, Ralph, & Scholz, Mark: *Invasion Of Prostate Snatchers: An Essential Guide To Managing Prostate CA For Patients And Their Families*

Recommended Websites:

http://pcai.pbworks.com

http://www.ustoo.org

www.mayoclinic.org

www.webmd.com

www.nafc.org

www.simonfoundation.org

Glossary of Surgeries and Treatments

•TURP (transurethral resection of the prostate): This is the most common surgery. An instrument is passed through the prostate and excess tissue is shaved off

•TUIP (transurethral incision of the prostate): Similar to TURP, a number of incisions are placed in the prostate to remove excessive tissue

•TUNA (transurethral needle ablation): Excess prostate tissue is burnt away using radio waves

•TUMT (transurethral microwave thermotherapy): Excess tissue is removed by microwaves sent through the catheter

•TUVP (transurethral electroevaporation of the prostate): An electrical current is used to vaporize excessive tissue

•Open prostatectomy; rarely performed nowadays—in this procedure the prostate is excised through an incision in the abdomen

Common Treatments for Prostate Cancer

Several options are available, including:

1. RALP: Robotic-assisted radical prostatectomy.

2. External beam radiation treatment: High energy X-Rays are beamed to the prostate from outside of the body.

3. Radioactive seed implants: Also known as brachytherapy, tiny radioactive "seeds" are implanted into the prostate gland.

4. Proton therapy: This involves positively charged particles radiated onto the prostate.

5. Watchful waiting.

6. High-intensity focused ultrasound or HIFU where ultrasound waves are beamed onto the prostate.

7. Laparoscopic prostatectomy: The prostate is removed through a small incision.

8. Radical perineal prostatectomy: The prostate is removed through the area between the rectum and scrotum.

9. Androgen deprivation therapy (ADT): Administered via injections as a chronic treatment.

10. Androgen therapy: Administered in the form of pills and in conjunction with other treatments.

Made in the USA
Monee, IL
26 February 2022

91914226R00118